S0-BCS-385

# PEDIATRIC NURSE PRACTITIONER

## *Certification Review*

### JoAnn Zerwekh, EdD, RN, FNP, CS
University of Phoenix
Carondelet Health Network Community Services
Tucson, Arizona
Nursing Education Consultants
Dallas, Texas

### Jo Carol Claborn, MS, RN, CNS
El Centro College
Nursing Education Consultants
Dallas, Texas

**W.B. SAUNDERS COMPANY**
*A Division of Harcourt Brace & Company*
Philadelphia    London    Toronto    Montreal    Sydney    Tokyo

**W.B. SAUNDERS COMPANY**
*A Division of Harcourt Brace & Company*

The Curtis Center
Independence Square West
Philadelphia, Pennsylvania 19106

**Library of Congress Cataloging-in-Publication Data**

Zerwekh, JoAnn Graham.
  Pediatric nurse practitioner certification review / JoAnn Zerwekh,
Jo Carol Claborn.
     p.   cm.
  ISBN 0–7216–7745–2
  1. Pediatric nursing—Examinations, questions, etc.  2. Nurse
practitioners—Examinations, questions, etc.  I. Claborn, Jo Carol.
II. Title.
  [DNLM:  1.  Pediatric Nursing examination questions.  2. Pediatric
Assessment examination questions.  3. Nursing process—
examination questions.  4. Nurse Practitioners examination
questions.  WY 18.2Z58p  1999]
DNLM/DLC                                                        99–28365

PEDIATRIC NURSE PRACTITIONER CERTIFICATION REVIEW  ISBN 0–7216–7745–2

Copyright © 1999 by W.B. Saunders Company

All rights reserved. No part of this publication may be reproduced or transmitted in any form or by any means, electronic or mechanical, including photocopy, recording, or any information storage and retrieval system, without permission in writing from the publisher.

Printed in the United States of America

Last digit is the print number:      9     8     7     6     5     4     3     2     1

*To Tom, my soul mate,*
*who brings a smile to my face and*
*a warm glow in my heart.*
*JoAnn*

*To Robert, my friend and partner,*
*whose love and patience keeps me going.*
*Jo*

# Series Contributors

Susan E. Chaney, EdD, MS, BSN
Professor, Family Nurse Practitioner
   Coordinator
Texas Woman's University
Family Nurse Practitioner
Homeless Outreach Medical Services
Parkland Health and Hospital System
Dallas, Texas

Cynthia Churgin, RN, FNP, CNM
Casa Blanca Medical Group
Mesa, Arizona

Sharon I. Decker, RN, CS, MSN,
   CCRN
Professor of Clinical Nursing
Director, Clinical Simulation Center
Texas Tech University Health Sciences
   Center
Lubbock, Texas

Nicolette Estrada, RN, MS, FNP-C
Chief Research Coordinator
Carl T. Hayden VA Medical Center
Phoenix, Arizona

Mary Jo Gagan, RNCS, FNP, PhD
Assistant Professor
University of Arizona College of Nursing
Nurse Practitioner
Campus Health
University of Arizona College of Nursing
Tucson, Arizona

Ela-Joy Lehrman, MS, MAEd, PhD
Program Manager for Nursing, Counseling,
   and General Studies
University of Phoenix
Tucson, Arizona

Beverly McCoy, BSN, MS, FNP
Clinical Director/Family Nurse Practitioner
Breaking the Circle Children's Health Care
Arizona State University
College of Nursing
Tempe, Arizona

Jacquelyn McGlamery, BSN, FNP
Family Nurse Practitioner
Sierra Tucson
Tucson, Arizona

Loretta Manning, RNC, MSN, GNP
Educational Consultant, Sylvia Rayfield &
   Associates
Executive Director, I CAN, Inc. Publishing
Atlanta, Georgia

Kathleen T. Ogle, RN, MS, CFNP
Instructor
Bowie State University
Department of Nursing
Bowie, Maryland;
Family Nurse Practitioner
Maryland Primary Care Physicians
Arnold, Maryland

Alice B. Pappas, BSN, MSN, PhD
Associate Dean for Academic Affairs
Baylor University School of Nursing
Dallas Texas

Jodi Pelusi, RN, MS, FNP
University of Phoenix
Phoenix, Arizona

Patricia J. Pinckard, MS, ANP
Adult Nurse Practitioner
Occupational Health
Desert Samaritan Medical Center
Mesa, Arizona

Sylvia M. Root, EdD, RNC, FNP
Associate Professor
Arizona State University
Tempe, Arizona

Patricia Scully, RN, MS, JD
Nurse Attorney Consultant
Tucson, Arizona

Patricia A. Shannon, RN, MS, CS, PNP
Faculty, University of Phoenix;
Director of Nurses and Nurse Practitioners
North Valley Pediatrics PC
Phoenix, Arizona;
Adjunct Faculty
Arizona State University
Tempe, Arizona;
President/Consultant
Pediatric Nursing . . . PLUS
Phoenix, Arizona

Linda Stevenson, RN, PhD
Baylor University School of Nursing
Dallas, Texas

Gail Tucker, RN, MS, FNP
BMT Nurse Practitioner
Good Samaritan Regional Medical Center;
City of Hope/Samaritan Bone Marrow
    Transplant
Phoenix, Arizona

Gayle P. Varnell, RN, CPNP, PhD
Assistant Professor
Nurse Practitioner Program Coordinator
The University of Texas at Tyler
Tyler, Texas

John Walter, RN, BS, CPNP
Guest Lecturer
Family Nurse Practitioner Program
University of Arizona College of Nursing;
Pediatric Nurse Practitioner
University Physicians
Tucson, Arizona

Pamela Becker Weilitz, AD, BSN,
    MSN(R)
Assistant Clinical Professor, Graduate
    Program
St. Louis University School of Nursing;
Adult Nurse Practitioner
Washington University School of Medicine
University Care
St. Louis, Missouri

Margaret "Pegi" Yancy, RN, MS,
    OGNP
Faculty Associate
Arizona State University
Tempe, Arizona;
Women's Health Nurse Practitioner
Department of Reproductive Medicine
St. Joseph's Hospital and Medical Center
Phoenix, Arizona

# Preface

With the dawn of the role of the nurse practitioner, there is an increasing need for additional reference information and study materials for the certification examinations. Nurse practitioners are playing a vital role in the changing health care delivery system in the United States. The numbers of candidates for the certification examinations is rapidly increasing as more nursing programs implement the nurse practitioner curriculum in their graduate programs. *Pediatric Nurse Practitioner Certification Review* has been developed to assist the advanced practice nurse to prepare for the PNP certification examination. Extensive efforts have been made to include current information that is representative of the content based on the blueprints for the certification exams. This book of questions is not intended to be an exhaustive review of the content, but an adjunct to the review process. Over 780 review questions are included in all.

Test-taking strategies are included in Chapter 1. As a candidate prepares for the examination, it is vitally important to be familiar with and to practice good testing strategies. Testing strategies can prevent the candidate from making mistakes and selecting the wrong answer. As the review process begins, a review of the testing strategies chapter and the practice of good testing strategies is critical. With many years experience in the field of testing, we have consistently identified the importance practice testing plays in the review process. Practice questions give the candidate an opportunity to review questions written from different perspectives. To enhance the review process, answers with complete rationales are provided at the end of each chapter. Not only does the candidate increase their knowledge of the subject area, but with more practice, testing skills become fine tuned. Good testing skills make the candidate more comfortable and help to decrease the stress associated with certification exams.

This book also includes chapters reviewing important concepts related to Growth and Development and Health Promotion and Maintenance. These chapters provide questions that test information related to growth and development, general health supervision, and health maintenance. The clinical chapters are developed using a systems approach, i.e., cardiovascular, respiratory, endocrine, etc. In each of these chapters, the test questions are divided into three areas: Physical Examination and Diagnostic Tests, Disorders, and Pharmacology. This format assists the candidate to easily locate specific questions. The last three chapters in the text are on Theory and Research; Issues and Trends; and Legal and Ethical aspects of nurse practitioner practice. The test questions in these chapters focus on professional competencies inherent in the role and function of the PNP.

Our thanks to the many nurse practitioners across the country who provided questions and insight into the role of the nurse practitioner. We wish to thank Robin Carter, our editor at W.B. Saunders, for her support and suggestions in our preparation of the manuscript. Thank you also goes to all the nurse practitioners who took time from their busy schedules to review the questions for content and clarity.

# Acknowledgments

W̶e are continually grateful for the contributions and efforts of our test item contributors who provided their expertise and knowledge for this nurse practitioner certification review series.

We thank the manuscript reviewers for their suggestions and insights as we tackled this large project:

Harvey Baker, RNCS, ARNP
Oswego Family Medical Clinic
Oswego, Kansas

Susan Appel, RN, MN, CCRN, CS
Carolinas College of Health
 Sciences
Charlotte, North Carolina

Genell Lee, BSN, MSN, JD
Hauth & Lee, LLC
Birmingham, Alabama

Stephanie A. Batalo, RN, BSN,
 MSN, FNP
Trinity Health System
Steubenville, Ohio

Dorothy J. Stuppy, RN, PhD
University of Texas at Arlington
Arlington, Texas

Lynette M. Wachholz, MN, RN,
 ARNP, IBCLC
The Everett Clinic
Everett, Washington

We thank the staff at W.B. Saunders Company: Robin Carter, Senior Editor, and Marie Pelcin and Ross Landy, editorial assistants for their calmness and patience. Joan Sinclair, who managed the book's production. It was such a pleasure to work with you again on another publication. Berta Steiner for copyediting and typesetting the manuscript. What a job to keep track of thousands of questions!

Last, but certainly not least, we want to thank: Our children, Tyler and Ashley Zerwekh, Jaelyn Claborn, Michael Brown, and Kim Aultman, for teasing their mothers about writing 5 books!! Our parents, Charles Graham and Hazel Cooper, for their continued support and encouragement. Tom Gaglione and Robert Claborn for their encouragement, support, and love. We love you all.

# Contents

# Test-Taking Strategies

## Testing Strategies

Knowing how to take an examination is a skill that is developed through practice and experience. Being able to take an examination effectively is almost as important as the basic knowledge required to answer the question. Everyone has taken an examination only to find in the review of the exam that questions were missed due to inadequate testing skills. Nurse practitioner programs provide the graduate student with a comprehensive base of knowledge; how you utilize this knowledge will determine your success on a certification examination. The certification examination is an objective test that covers knowledge, understanding, and application of professional nursing theory and practice. When you register for the examination, you will receive a "Candidate Handbook" or information materials from the Certification Board administering the examination. This handbook will have helpful information to assist you in preparing, such as important registration information, test content outline, sample test questions, and in some cases a bibliography. This important information can assist you in your review process.

Read the information in this chapter carefully and make sure you understand the strategies discussed. This chapter is designed to help you identify problem areas in testing skills and learn how to use strategy and judgment in selecting correct answers. It is important for you to practice test-ing skills if you are going to be able to utilize these skills on the certification examination.

## Question Characteristics

A. Multiple-choice questions.
  1. Scene or scenario—establishes the setting of the question. Not all questions will have a scenario; if a scenario is included, consider the appropriateness of the answer to the information provided.
  2. Stem—states the question that is being asked.
  3. Options—there are four options from which to choose an answer.
     a. Distractors—designed to distract you from the correct answer.
     b. Correct answer—correctly answers the question asked in the stem.
     c. There are only four options in any item; there are no combinations of options to consider.
     d. There is only one correct response; no partial credit is given for another answer.
B. Questions are derived from clinical situations common in the practice setting.

# Strategies for Multiple-Choice Questions

**1. Cover the options with your hand or a piece of scratch paper.**\* This strategy makes you focus on the content of the question and prevents your eyes from "darting" to look at the distractors. If you peruse the distractors before you completely understand the question, key words in the distractors will influence your interpretation of the question.

**2. Do not read extra meaning into the question.** The question is asking for specific information; if it appears to be simple "common sense," then assume it is simple. Do not look for a hidden meaning in what appears to be an easy question.

### E X A M P L E :

A 2-year-old Asian-American child comes to the clinic with her parents and infant brother. The chief complaint is abdominal pain, flatulence, and diarrhea after eating. Until 3 months ago, she had continued to be breast-fed twice a day. The nurse practitioner would suspect:

1. Irritable bowel syndrome.
2. Hirschsprung's disease.
3. Lactose intolerance.
4. Food allergy.

*The correct answer is Option #3. Be careful to not "read into" the question and make the child have a more serious disorder. Lactose intolerance is common among Asian clients. The primary symptoms are bloating, flatulence, abdominal cramps, and diarrhea for 2 hours after lactose-containing food consumption.*

### E X A M P L E :

When administering skin tests to an immunocompromised child, the nurse practitioner must consider:

1. The importance of not applying more than one skin test at a time.
2. The skin test may react more aggressively than expected.
3. The use of a known allergen for the client and utilize it as a control.
4. The immunocompromised client should not be skin tested.

*The correct answer is Option #3. Do not read into the question and make it more difficult by trying to make the client sicker (i.e., full-blown acquired immunodeficiency syndrome [AIDS]). It is important to remember to apply controls when skin testing the immunocompromised client. Ask clients what diseases they believe they have immunity to, such as measles. Apply the "known" allergen and the skin test to be tested. If the client is unable to mount an immune response at all, the known allergen will not react. By not applying the controls, the nurse practitioner may assume a skin test is negative, when in fact the client's immune system is unable to respond.*

**3. Read the stem correctly.** Make sure you understand exactly what information the question is asking.

### E X A M P L E :

The nurse practitioner would refer to a pediatric cardiologist, for work-up and evaluation within 1–2 weeks, a child with:

1. Signs of exercise intolerance, dyspnea, and elevated pulse.
2. Poor feeding, increased cyanosis with crying, and dizziness.
3. Nonfunctional heart murmur, respiratory crackles, and retarded growth and development.
4. Systolic ejection murmur, grade II which disappears on sitting.

*The question asks you to determine which child's symptoms would require a referral to a pediatric cardiologist within the next 1–2 weeks. Options #1, #2, and #3 are considered unstable and acute and should be immediately referred to a pediatric cardiologist. Children with a murmur need to be further evaluated, but it is not considered an emergency as long as they are asymptomatic, have normal activity and exercise, and are growing normally.*

**4. Before considering the options, formulate in your mind possible answers to the question.** If none of the options fit in the pool of answers you anticipated, go back and re-evaluate the question. Assess each of the options with regard to your pool of possible answers.

---

\*This testing strategy of covering the distractors is from Phoebe K. Helm, Ed.D.

**EXAMPLE:**

The nurse practitioner is assessing a child with a history of a patent ductus arteriosus. What symptoms are characteristic of this condition?

1. Cyanosis that is noted on exertion and when child is crying.
2. Child assumes a squatting position when playing.
3. Child has increased difficulty breathing with activity, but no cyanosis.
4. Tachycardia and cyanosis occur with minimal amount of physical exertion.

*Formulate in your mind possible answers. Think to yourself, "What is typically found in a child with PDA? Are there respiratory problems? Do these children get cyanotic or not?" PDA is an acyanotic condition. Squatting along with finger clubbing occurs with cyanotic conditions. Option #3 is the correct answer.*

**5. Identify what type of response the question is asking for.** A positive stem requires identification of three false items and one true item as the correct answer.

**EXAMPLE:**

Adolescents who believe they have been exposed to human immunodeficiency virus (HIV) should have an HIV antibody test how soon after the exposure?

1. The next day and 2 months later.
2. 6 months after exposure and again at 12 months.
3. 6–12 weeks after exposure and again at 6 months.
4. 4 weeks and 12 weeks.

*The correct answer is Option #3. This question requires you to identify three incorrect responses and one correct response. The HIV antibody develops between 6 and 12 weeks after exposure. Because of the variability of antibody development, it is recommended that the test be repeated in 6 months to confirm the findings.*

**6. Identify questions that require identification of something the practitioner should not or would not do (i.e., unsafe action, contraindication, inappropriate action).**

**EXAMPLE:**

The practitioner is prescribing astemizole (Hismanal) for an older adolescent's allergy problems. When considering the adolescent's current medications, which medication would be a contraindication to the administration of astemizole (Hismanal)?

1. Erythromycin ethylsuccinate (E.E.S.)
2. Tetracycline (Achromycin).
3. Amoxicillin (Amoxil).
4. Trimethoprim-sulfamethoxazole (Bactrim).

*The correct answer is Option #1. Macrolides and Hismanal should not be administered concurrently. The nurse practitioner is required to identify a medication that should not be ordered.*

**7. Questions may also be analytical.** These questions may ask the nurse practitioner to identify findings, statements, and the like that are consistent/inconsistent with the client's presenting problem and/or differentiate between them.

**EXAMPLE:**

A child is being evaluated for attention deficit hyperactivity disorder (ADHD). Which test is helpful in evaluating the difference between ADHD and a learning disability?

1. Standardized IQ achievement test.
2. Denver Developmental Screening Test.
3. Audiological and visual testing.
4. Complete neurologic examination.

*Before you examine the options in this question, it is important to think about the differences between ADHD and learning disabilities. The correct answer is Option #1. Children with learning disabilities and ADHD are often impulsive, inattentive, and overactive. Usually, children with ADHD do not have lower IQ achievement scores; however, children with a learning disability usually demonstrate a level of educational achievement substantially below that of the IQ.*

**8. Identify key words that affect your understanding of the question.** Make sure you understand exactly what information the question is asking. Be aware of questions in which the stem includes words such as *except, contraindicated, avoid, least, not applicable,* and *does not occur.* These words change the direction of the question. It may help to rephrase the question in your own words in order to better understand what information is being requested.

---

**E X A M P L E :**

---

Anticipatory guidance for the family of a 9-month-old includes all **except**:

1. Use of shoes for protection, not support.
2. Encourage self-feeding.
3. Baby-proof home; pool and water safety.
4. Issues of independence and dependence.

*It is helpful to rephrase the question: What is important guidance to teach the family of a 9-month-old? It is important that you identify the key point "anticipatory guidance of a 9-month-old" and the key word "except." If you miss these essential points, you do not understand the question, and chances are you will not choose the correct answer. The correct answer is Option #4. Issues of independence and dependence are usually discussed with the parents of a 2-year-old. All of the other options are appropriate for anticipatory guidance of a 9-month-old, along with talking to the child and avoiding bottle tooth decay (no bottle in the bed).*

---

**9. As you read the options, eliminate those you know are not correct.** This will help narrow the field of choice. When you select an answer or eliminate a distractor, you should have a specific reason for doing so.

---

**E X A M P L E :**

---

In an event where a knee "gives out," usually associated with trauma, followed by severe pain and effusion and later "locking" of the knee with pivoting or turning, the adolescent has probably suffered:

1. Patellofemoral stress syndrome. (*No, there is a dull, aching pain with some clicking; long periods of sitting or activities that involve knee flexion as well as compression of the patella in the groove cause increased pain.*)
2. Growing pains. (*No, the pain usually occurs at night and resolves by morning; the pain is deep and does not involve the joints.*)
3. Shin splints. (*No, inflammation of muscles along the medial shaft of the tibia due to overuse causes aching pain and rest improves the pain; improper warm-up exercises can lead to the pain.*)

4. Patellar subluxation. (*Yes, the knee "gives out" and the patella is laterally displaced, with severe pain and an effusion and subsequent "locking" of the knee with pivoting or turning.*)

*The correct answer is Option #4.*

---

**10. Identify similarities in the distractors.** Frequently, three distractors will contain similar information, and one will be different. The different one may be the correct answer.

---

**E X A M P L E :**

---

A mother is encouraged to increase the protein in her child's diet. The addition of which of these foods to 100 ml of milk will provide the greatest amount of protein?

1. 50 ml light cream and 2 tbsp corn syrup.
2. 30 gm powdered skim milk and one egg.
3. 1 small scoop (90 gm) ice cream and 1 tbsp chocolate syrup.
4. 2 egg yolks and 1 tbsp sugar.

*Options #1, #3, and #4 all contain a simple sugar. The correct answer, Option #2, has more protein. Notice that three of the options are similar; the one that is different may be the correct answer. This strategy is not a substitute for basic knowledge but may help you figure out the answer.*

---

**11. Select the most comprehensive answer.** All of the options may be correct, but **one** will include the other three options or need to be considered first.

---

**E X A M P L E :**

---

A new mother tells the nurse practitioner that her infant was born HIV-positive. She asks the nurse practitioner how long her baby has to live. The nurse practitioner's response would be based on the knowledge that:

1. The antibodies present in the baby's blood may reflect the antibodies received from the mother at the time of birth.
2. If antibodies are present at birth, the baby has AIDS in an active form.
3. Since the baby is HIV-positive, the child will develop full-blown AIDS within 3 years.
4. The antibodies detected at birth indicate presence of the HIV; the test does not indicate when the child will develop AIDS.

*The correct answer is Option #4. It is important to give the mother as much hope as possible but still be realistic about the condition. There is no way to tell when or if the child will convert to active AIDS. Many infants seroconvert to HIV-negative status.*

**12. Select the best answer that is most specific to what the question asks.** All of the options may be correct, but **one** is more specific or essential.

**E X A M P L E :**

When a child comes in for a health maintenance clinic visit, what is essential for the nurse practitioner to do?

1. Order routine laboratory tests.
2. Perform vision and auditory screening.
3. Plot height and weight on charts.
4. Review immunization record.

*It is absolutely essential that the immunization record be reviewed. The other options are important but are not essential for a health maintenance visit. Recognize key words that identify the question that is asking for a priority of care—first, initial, best, most. The correct answer is Option #4; the other alternatives may be correct but should be prioritized.*

**13. Watch questions in which the options contain several items to consider.** After you are sure you understand what information the question is requesting, evaluate each part of the option. Is it appropriate to what the question is asking? If an option contains one incorrect item, the entire option is incorrect. All of the items listed in the selection must be correct, if it is to be the answer to the question.

**E X A M P L E :**

The nurse practitioner suspects drug use in an adolescent. Physical findings of cocaine abuse include:

1. Bradycardia, miosis, hypertension.
2. Hypertension, tachycardia, tremor.
3. Hypotension, bradycardia, abdominal cramps.
4. Decreased level of consciousness, tachycardia, excessive salivation.

*The correct answer is Option #2. In a methodical evaluation of the items in the distractors, you can eliminate certain items in Option #1 (bradycardia), Option #3 (bradycardia and hypotension), and Option #4 (excessive salivation). Bradycardia, hypotension, and excessive salivation are not found with cocaine abuse.*

**14. Be alert to relevant information contained in previous questions.** Sometimes, as you are answering questions, you will find information similar to the question being tested. Previous questions may assist you to identify relevant information in the current question.

**E X A M P L E :**

Before giving a child the measles-mumps-rubella (MMR) trivalent vaccine, it is recommended to wait how long after chemotherapy has stopped?

1. 30 days.
2. 2 months.
3. 3 months.
4. 6 months.

*The correct answer is Option #3. The MMR is a live-virus vaccine, and children severely immunosuppressed due to cancer therapy should not be given a live-virus vaccine until immunoglobulin levels have increased, or they will be at increased risk for serious complications and the disease. In another question involving immunizations, you read the following question:*

**E X A M P L E :**

The nurse practitioner understands that the following is considered an attenuated live-virus vaccination:

1. Rubella and measles.
2. Mumps and hepatitis B.
3. Poliomyelitis and hepatitis B.
4. Rubella and rabies.

*The correct answer is Option #1. A clue to the answer to this question may be found in the previous question—the MMR is a live-virus vaccine. Attenuated live-virus vaccines are available for the following communicable diseases: measles, mumps, rubella, poliomyelitis, yellow fever, and smallpox. Rabies vaccine is a killed virus and hepatitis B is a purified viral antigen obtained from the blood of an infected client and then inactivated when manufactured into a vaccine.*

**15. Multiple-choice mathematical computations may be included in the exam.** Mathematical computations may include calculations of IM, PO, and IV dosages; calculations of pediatric dosage; determining creatinine clearance; and conversion of units of measurement.

### E X A M P L E :

The nurse practitioner is ordering amoxicillin (Amoxil) for a child with otitis media. The child weighs 22 lbs. How would the order be written?

1. Amoxicillin 250 mg/5 ml Sig: 5 ml PO tid × 10 days.
2. Amoxicillin 500 mg Sig: 1 tab PO tid × 3 days.
3. Amoxicillin 350 mg/5 ml Sig: 5 ml PO bid × 14 days.
4. Amoxicillin 125 mg/5 ml Sig: 5 ml PO tid × 10 days.

*First, you must convert the lbs to kgs, which is 2.2 lbs/kg. This child weighs 10 kg. The dose for amoxicillin is 30–50 mg/kg/day for a child. 10 kg × 40 mg/kg/day = 400 mg/day. Amoxicillin is supplied in 125 mg/5 ml and 250 mg/5 ml. The correct dose for this child would be the 125 mg/5 ml. The answer closest to that dosage is Option #4.*

**16. Evaluate priority questions carefully. Frequently all of the answers are appropriate to the situation.** You need to decide which of the actions you should do first.

### E X A M P L E :

While attending a rural public school, a 7-year-old child was bitten on the hand by a raccoon. At the rural clinic, the nurse practitioner cleansed the wound. The next action is:

1. Administer tetanus antitoxin.
2. Contact local animal control authorities.
3. Administer rabies immune globulin (RIG) and human diploid cell vaccine (HDCV).
4. Teach the family how to do hourly soaks to the hand using normal saline and peroxide.

*The correct answer is Option #3. Any type of animal bite that might be associated with an animal that may potentially harbor rabies (skunks, bats, raccoons, foxes, coyotes, rats) should be treated with both active and passive rabies immunization. The priority action is to prevent rabies. Tetanus antitoxin would be indicated if the child was not current on the immunization. Animal authorities would be called after the initial treatment to locate the animal and sacrifice it, so that the brain can be examined for rabies.*

## Techniques to Increase Critical Thinking Skills

Memory aids and mindmapping are tools that assist in drawing associations from other ideas with the use of visual images. Mnemonics are words, phrases, or other techniques that help you remember information. Imagery is a tool that helps you identify a problem and visualize a mental picture. Learning content utilizing these techniques will assist you to recall information more effectively.

**Mindmapping**™ is a method of organizing important information that is in sharp contrast to the traditional outline format. A thought or concept is written in the center of the page, and images and color are added to information as ideas begin to flow from the center focus (see Fig. 1–1).

**Acronyms** assist you to recall information via word association or arrangements of letters to recall specific information. Examples of these are: BRAT Diet (see Fig. 1–2), 6-Ps of dyspnea (see Fig. 1–3), the 5-Ps of circulatory assessment (see Fig. 1–4), and the ABCs of malignant melanoma (see Fig. 1–5).

**Acrostics** are catchy phrases in which the first letter of each word stands for something to recall. For example, in remembering the use of canes and walkers (Fig. 1–6) think of "Wandering Wilma's Always Late" (**W**alker **W**ith **A**ffected **L**eg). Everyone remembers the cranial nerve mnemonic (see Fig. 1–7).

**Memory aids or images** are pictures or caricatures that help you to recall information more effectively (see Fig. 1–8).

**Rhymes** are phrases or words spoken in a rhythmical or musical manner that increase recall. A helpful musical rhyme for hypoglycemia versus hyperglycemia is "hot and dry, sugar high; cold and clammy, need some candy" (see Fig. 1–9). Another rhyme, "fingers, nose, penis, toes," identifies the areas where lidocaine with epinephrine is contraindicated as a local anesthetic. Or, "two is too much" may help you remember toxic levels of the following three drugs, which have a narrow margin of safety—lithium, digoxin, theophylline (see Fig. 1–10).

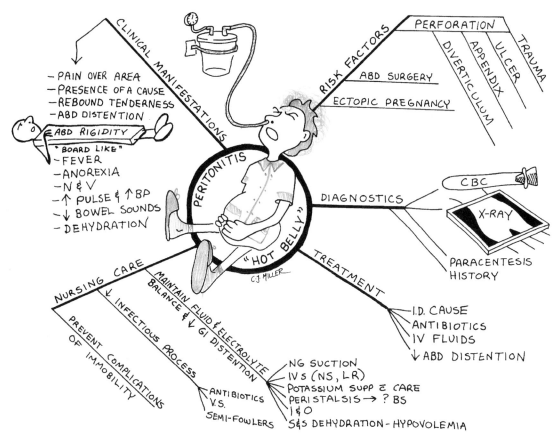

**FIGURE 1–1**  PERITONITIS "HOT BELLY"
From Zerwekh J, Claborn J, Miller CJ: Memory Notebook of Nursing, Vol I. Dallas, TX: Nursing Education Consultants Publishing, Inc, 1994, p. 85, with permission.

*Note: These are just examples. There are entire books on these helpful aids (see the list of references).*

## Testing Skills for Paper-and-Pencil Tests

1. Go through the exam and mark all the answers that you know are correct. This ensures you have adequate time to answer the questions you know. Go back and evaluate those questions for which you did not readily recognize the answer.

2. Do not indiscriminately change answers. If you go back and change an answer, you should have a specific reason for doing so. Sometimes you remember information and realize you answered the question incorrectly. Frequently, test-takers "talk themselves out of" the correct answer and change it to an incorrect one.

3. After you have completed the exam, go back and check your booklet and make sure all of the questions are answered. Answer all of the questions, even if you must guess.

## Testing Skills that Apply to Both Paper-and-Pencil Tests and Computer Testing

1. Listen carefully to the instructions given at the beginning of the examination. Make sure you understand all of the information given and exactly how to mark your answers, and/or how to use the keyboard.

2. Watch your timing. Do not spend too much time on one question. It is very important that you practice your timing on the sample exams. When you begin to take a paper-and-pencil test, plan on finishing within the first three fourths of the allocated time. It is not necessary to review all of the questions after

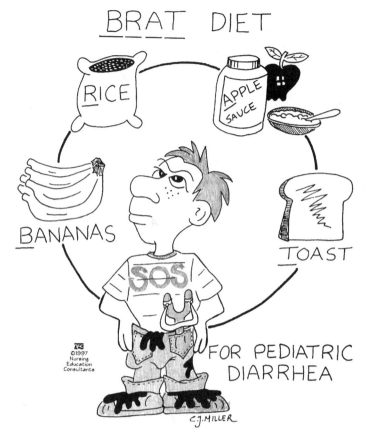

**FIGURE 1–2**   BRAT DIET
From Zerwekh J, Claborn J, Miller CJ: Memory Notebook of Nursing, Vol II. Dallas, TX: Nursing Education Consultants Publishing, Inc, 1997, p. 17, with permission.

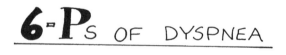

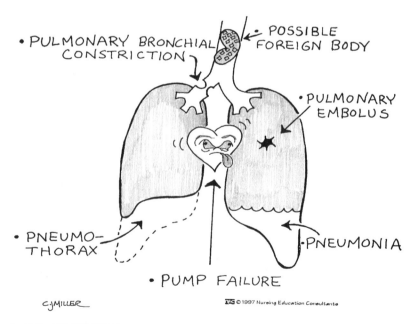

**FIGURE 1–3**   6-Ps OF DYSPNEA
From Zerwekh J, Claborn J, Miller CJ: Memory Notebook of Nursing, Vol II. Dallas, TX: Nursing Education Consultants Publishing, Inc, 1997, p. 22, with permission.

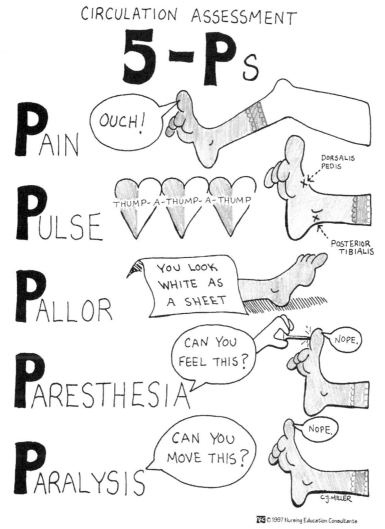

**FIGURE 1–4**  CIRCULATION ASSESSMENT: THE 5-Ps
From Zerwekh J, Claborn J, Miller CJ: Memory Notebook of Nursing, Vol II. Dallas, TX: Nursing Education Consultants Publishing, Inc, 1997, p. 27, with permission.

you have completed the test. Do it right the first time and there is no need to review the entire test again. Go back and answer the questions that you left blank. Watch your timing on computer tests—make use of a computer clock, if it is available.

3. Be aware of your "first hunch." It is frequently the correct answer. Sometimes information is processed by the brain without you being aware of it. If something about an answer "feels right" or you have a "gut-level feeling," pay attention to it.

4. Eliminate distractors that assume the client "would not understand," or "is ignorant" of the situation, or those that "protect them from worry." For example, "The client should

not be told she has cancer because it would upset her too much."

5. Be aware of distractors that contain the words *always* and *never*.

6. There is no pattern of correct answers. Both computer and paper-and-pencil examinations are compiled by a computer, and the position of the correct answers is selected at random.

## Decrease Anxiety

Your activities the day of the examination strongly influence your level of anxiety. By care-

# HINTS TO MALIGNANT MELANOMA

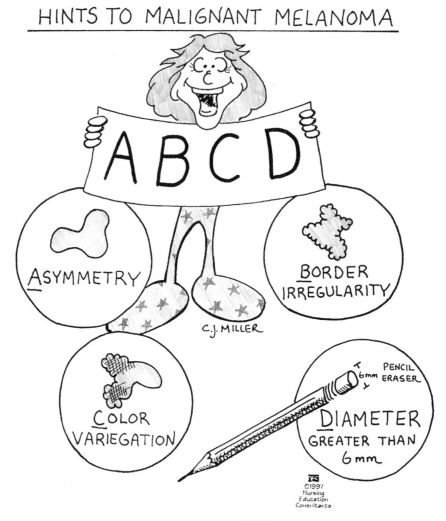

**FIGURE 1–5**  HINTS TO MALIGNANT MELANOMA (ABCD)
From Zerwekh J, Claborn J, Miller CJ: Memory Notebook of Nursing, Vol II. Dallas, TX: Nursing Education Consultants Publishing, Inc, 1997, p. 137, with permission.

fully planning ahead, you will be able to eliminate some anxiety-provoking situations. If you are a diabetic or have special needs, contact the certification agency ahead of time to make arrangements to have food or other accommodations that you might require.

1. Visit the examination site prior to the day of the exam. Evaluate travel time, parking, and time to get to the designated area. Get an early start to allow extra time.

2. If you must travel some distance to the examination site, plan to spend the night in the immediate vicinity.

3. Do something pleasant the evening prior to the examination. This is not the time to "crash study."

4. Anxiety is contagious. If those around you are extremely anxious, avoid contact with them prior to the examination.

5. Make your meal before the test a light, healthy one.

6. Avoid eating highly spiced or different foods. This is not the time for a gastrointestinal upset.

7. Wear comfortable clothes. This is not a good time to wear tight clothing or new shoes.

8. Wear clothing of moderate weight. It is difficult to control the temperature to keep everyone comfortable. Take a sweater or wear layered clothes that can be removed if you get too warm.

9. Wear soft-soled shoes; this decreases the noise in the testing area.

10. Make sure you have the papers that are required to gain admission to the exam site. Do not forget your reading glasses, if you wear them.

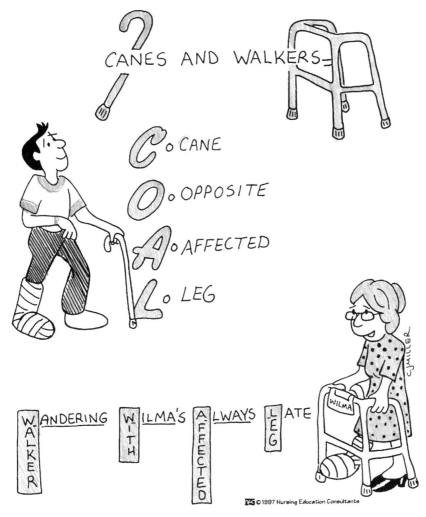

**FIGURE 1–6**   CANES AND WALKERS

From Zerwekh J, Claborn J, Miller CJ: Memory Notebook of Nursing, Vol II. Dallas, TX: Nursing Education Consultants Publishing, Inc, 1997, p. 8, with permission.

11. Do not take study material to the exam site. You cannot take it into the exam area and it is too late to study.

12. Do not panic when you encounter content with which you are unfamiliar in a question. Use good test-taking strategies, select an answer, and continue. Remember, you are not going to know all of the right answers.

13. Reaffirm to yourself that you know the material. It is not time for any self-defeating behavior or negative self-talk. **YOU WILL PASS!!** Build your confidence by visualizing yourself in 6 months working in the area you desire. Create that mental picture of where you want to be and who you want to be—certified nurse practitioner. Use your past successes to bring positive energy

and "vibes" to your certification. **WE KNOW YOU CAN DO IT!**

## Study Habits

### *Enhancing Study Skills*

- Decide on a study schedule—write it down and stick with it.
- Divide the review material into segments —pediatric acute illness, growth and development, and so forth.
- Prioritize the segments; review first the areas in which you feel you are deficient and/or weak.

# CRANIAL NERVE MNEMONIC

| S = Sensory | M = Motor | B = Both |
|---|---|---|

| | | | | | | | |
|---|---|---|---|---|---|---|---|
| O | Olfactory | O | On | S | Some | | |
| O | Optic | O | Old | S | Say | | |
| O | Oculomotor | O | Olympus' | M | Marry | | |
| T | Trochlear | T | Tiny | M | Money | | |
| T | Trigeminal | T | Tops | B | But | | |
| A | Abducens | A | A | M | My | | |
| F | Facial | F | Finn | B | Brother | | |
| A | Acoustic | A | And | S | Says | | |
| G | Glossopharyngeal | G | German | B | Bad | | |
| V | Vagus nerve | V | Viewed | B | Business | | |
| S | Spinal | S | Some | M | Marry | | |
| H | Hypoglossal | H | Hops | M | Money | | |

© 1994 Nursing Education Consultants

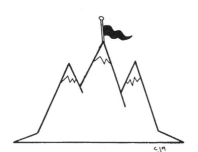 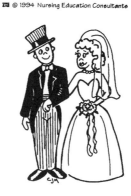

**FIGURE 1–7**   CRANIAL NERVE MNEMONIC
From Zerwekh J, Claborn J, Miller CJ: Memory Notebook of Nursing, Vol I. Dallas, TX: Nursing Education Consultants Publishing, Inc, 1994, p. 91, with permission.

## HYPERTHYROIDISM

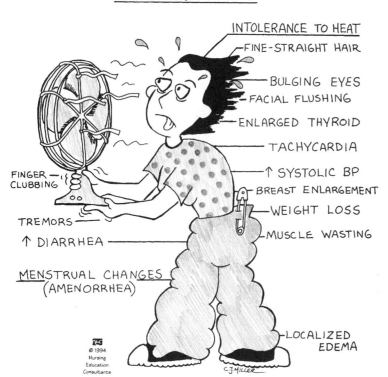

INTOLERANCE TO HEAT
FINE-STRAIGHT HAIR
BULGING EYES
FACIAL FLUSHING
ENLARGED THYROID
TACHYCARDIA
↑ SYSTOLIC BP
BREAST ENLARGEMENT
WEIGHT LOSS
MUSCLE WASTING
FINGER CLUBBING
TREMORS
↑ DIARRHEA
MENSTRUAL CHANGES (AMENORRHEA)
LOCALIZED EDEMA
© 1994 Nursing Education Consultants
C.J. MILLER

**FIGURE 1–8**   HYPERTHYROIDISM
From Zerwekh J, Claborn J, Miller CJ: Memory Notebook of Nursing, Vol I. Dallas, TX: Nursing Education Consultants Publishing, Inc, 1994, p. 46, with permission.

# BLOOD SUGAR MNEMONIC

## Hot & Dry = Sugar High

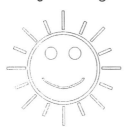

## Cold & Clammy = Need Some Candy

**FIGURE 1–9**  BLOOD SUGAR MNEMONIC
From Zerwekh J, Claborn J, Miller CJ: Memory Notebook of Nursing, Vol I. Dallas, TX: Nursing Education Consultants Publishing, Inc, 1994, p. 50, with permission.

- Identify areas that will require additional review.
- Establish a realistic schedule—study in short segments or "bursts." Avoid marathon sessions.
- Plan on achieving your study goal several days prior to the examination.
- Do not study when you are tired or when there are frequent distractions or interruptions.
- Review general concepts of practice from a variety of resources.

### Group Study

- Keep the group limited to four or five people.
- Group members should be mature and serious about studying.
- The group should agree on the planned study schedule.
- If the group makes you anxious or you do not feel it meets your study needs, do not continue to participate.

### Testing Practice

- Include the testing practice in your schedule.
- Select about 50 questions for a practice testing session of 1 hour. This will allow you to evaluate the pace of the exam (i.e., approximately a question per minute).
- Try to answer the questions as if you were taking the real examination. Do not look up the right answer immediately after answering the question.
- Utilize the testing strategies described in this chapter.
- Evaluate the practice exams for problem areas: testing skills and knowledge base.
- Evaluate the questions you answer incorrectly. Review the rationale for the right answer and understand why you missed it.
- Utilize the questions at a later point to review the information again.

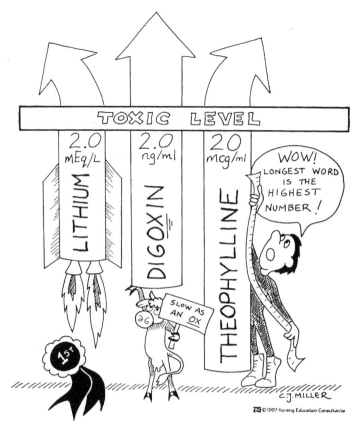

**FIGURE 1–10**  TOXIC LEVELS OF LITHIUM, DIGOXIN, AND THEOPHYLLINE
From Zerwekh J, Claborn J, Miller CJ: Memory Notebook of Nursing, Vol II. Dallas, TX: Nursing Education Consultants Publishing, Inc, 1997, p. 43, with permission.

## References

Beitz J: Unleashing the power of memory: The mighty mnemonic. *Nurse Educator*, 22(2), 25–28, 1997.

Bloomingfield R: Mnemonics, Rhetorics, and Poetics for Medics. Salem, NC: Harbinger Medical Press, 1982.

Rayfield S, Manning L: Nursing Made Insanely Easy. Shreveport, LA: ICAN, Inc. Publishing, 1997.

Zerwekh J, Claborn J: Test-taking strategies. In NCLEX-RN™: A comprehensive study guide, 3rd ed. Dallas, TX: Nursing Education Consultants Publishing, Inc, 1997.

Zerwekh J, Claborn J, Miller CJ: Memory Notebook of Nursing, Vol I. Dallas, TX: Nursing Education Consultants Publishing, Inc, 1994.

Zerwekh J, Claborn J, Miller CJ: Memory Notebook of Nursing, Vol II. Dallas, TX: Nursing Education Consultants Publishing, Inc, 1997.

# 2

# Growth & Development

## Physical Assessment

1. The following is the sequence recommended for well-child examinations up to the age of 5:

   1. 2 weeks, 2 months, 4 months, 6 months, 1 year, 15 months, 18 months, and every year from age 2 to age 5.

   2. 2 months, 4 months, 6 months, 9 months, annually from years 1 to 5.

   3. 2 weeks, 2 months, 4 months, 6 months, 9 months, 12 months, 15 months, 18 months, and annually years 2 to 5.

   4. The same intervals recommended for immunizations.

2. An appropriate treatment for overweight children under 8 years of age would include:

   1. Administer an appetite suppressant.

   2. Eliminate all carbohydrates in the diet.

   3. Plan a program of activity and exercise.

   4. Use vitamin therapy and herbal teas.

3. The nurse practitioner is seeing a 2-week-old newborn on the first clinic visit. She notes dysmorphic facial features. The nurse practitioner's evaluation includes:

   1. Ordering a chromosome analysis.

   2. Complete postnatal history.

   3. Detailed physical examination and perinatal history.

   4. Avoiding discussion with parents until diagnostic studies are completed.

4. An 18-month-old's feet turn inward. The mother is concerned; however, the child is unaware of it. The differential diagnosis includes all **except**:

   1. Femoral anteversion.

   2. Metatarsus adductus.

   3. Legg-Calvé-Perthes disease.

   4. Adducted great toe.

5. The characteristics of an innocent heart murmur in children include:

   1. Asymptomatic, loud diastolic rumble, grade IV.

   2. Midsystolic, no thrill, and asymptomatic.

   3. Asymptomatic with an $S_4$ heard at left lower sternal border (LSB).

   4. May disappear on sitting and following any type of physical activity.

6. The nurse practitioner is examining a 6-month-old infant. What would be the anticipated findings on examining the infant's fontanels?

   1. Both anterior and posterior should be open.

   2. The anterior should be open, the posterior closed.

   3. Both anterior and posterior should be closed.

   4. The anterior should be closed, the posterior open.

7. Genu varum up to 20 degrees is normal until age:

   1. 18 years old.

   2. 5 years old.

   3. 18 months old.

   4. 6 months old.

8. When approaching a toddler to complete a cardiac assessment, the nurse practitioner would:

   1. Allow the toddler to handle the stethoscope while the history is being taken.

   2. Explain in detail what you are going to do and the get toddler involved.

   3. Keep the child warm and covered to minimize discomfort.

   4. Approach the child by cheerfully calling his name out.

9. In performing a physical examination, the nurse practitioner first allows the child to touch the medical equipment and then begins by examining the extremities. This

sequence would be most appropriate to use for what age client?

   1. Infant.

   2. Toddler.

   3. School-age child.

   4. Adolescent.

10. An appropriate test to do to check for color perception in a preschooler would be:

    1. Ishihara's test.

    2. Bruchner's test.

    3. Hirschberg's test.

    4. Jaeger's test.

11. When assessing the cranial nerves in a young child, the nurse practitioner should:

    1. Obtain help from the parents to enlist the child's cooperation.

    2. Defer assessing the cranial nerves until the child is older.

    3. Modify the technique of examination based on the child's developmental level.

    4. Expect minimal variations among age groups.

12. The nurse practitioner understands the following about the Denver Developmental Screening Test–Revised (DDST-R or Denver II):

    1. It is a measurement of intelligence (IQ).

    2. It screens personal/social, fine and gross motor, and language skills.

    3. It is conducted when the examiner pronounces words and the child repeats.

    4. It is used for ages 0–36 months.

13. Genu valgum is considered normal from:

    1. 1–2 years old.

    2. 2–6 years old.

    3. 8–10 years old.

    4. 12–16 years old.

14. An African-American mother and her newborn are seen by the nurse practitioner for a well-baby visit. The mother is responsive to the baby's cries, and the baby comforts easily and makes frequent eye contact with the mother. Upon examination, the nurse practitioner notes the following: height and weight are at the 75th percentile on growth charts, there is a strong sucking reflex, and there is a large blue-black macular lesion over the lumbosacral area. The nurse practitioner should:

    1. Contact a social worker and report the mother to Child Protective Services immediately.

    2. Refer the mother and infant to a dermatologist.

    3. Recognize that the blue-black spot is a Mongolian spot, and counsel the mother that no treatment is necessary.

    4. Prescribe clotrimazole cream 1% (Mycelex) bid for 4 weeks.

15. The plantar fat pad, which makes a young child appear to have pes planus, is normal until age:

    1. 1–2 years old.

    2. 2–3 years old.

    3. 2–6 years old.

    4. 6–8 years old.

16. Growth hormone secretion tests along with a history and physical exam have indicated a positive diagnosis for delayed puberty. The next step for the nurse practitioner is to:

    1. Treat with hormone replacement.

    2. Refer to pediatric endocrinologist.

    3. Treat with hormone stimulation therapy.

    4. Refer for possible pituitary tumor.

17. During the physical examination of a 13-year-old female, it is developmentally important that the nurse practitioner:

    1. Maintain a comfortable silence.

    2. Verbally affirm normalcy.

    3. Discuss only the major areas of abnormality.

    4. Verbally address problems of sexually transmitted diseases.

18. At a school clinic a 14-year-old girl comes in complaining of dizziness midmorning and a second episode in class later in the morning. The practitioner should question the adolescent regarding diet/nutrition, drug use, and:

    1. Asthma.

    2. Pregnancy.

    3. Heart disease.

    4. Stress.

19. The nurse practitioner understands that sulfa medications are not recommended for children less than which age?

    1. 18 months.

    2. 12 months.

    3. 6 months.

    4. 2 months.

## Growth & Development

20. The major influence on the timing of puberty is:

    1. Exposure to light.

    2. Genetics.

    3. General health.

    4. Nutrition.

21. A 14-year-old girl is seen in the clinic by the nurse practitioner because she has not achieved menarche. Examination reveals axillary and pubic hair and breast buds with increased size of areola. Based on these findings the most appropriate intervention would be:

    1. Bone age studies.

    2. Labs for luteinizing hormone (LH) and follicle-stimulating hormone (FSH) levels.

    3. Chromosome analysis to rule out Turner's syndrome.

    4. Reassurance that she is developing normally.

22. A 13-year-old male is seen by the nurse practitioner for a sports physical. The genital exam reveals straight dark pubic hair at the base of the penis and testicular enlargement. Using the Tanner scale, the practitioner would record these findings as:

    1. Tanner stage I. → ∅   *pubic Hair*
    2. Tanner stage II. → *Countable, straight, ↑ pig + length*
    3. Tanner stage III. → *Darker, begin to curl, ↑ quantity*
    4. Tanner stage IV. → *↑ quantity, cover most pubic area*
    V → *Adult distribution, spread to lower thighs and lower abdomen*

23. An 11-year-old girl who has just begun to show signs of breast development asks the nurse practitioner when she will start having periods like her friends. The practitioner's response is based on the knowledge that:

    1. The average age of menarche is 12.8 years.
    2. Most girls will have a growth spurt following the onset of menarche.
    3. Menarche usually occurs about 3–6 months after the onset of breast development.
    4. Menarche usually occurs about 18–24 months after the onset of breast development.

24. A teenage girl with curly pubic hair on the mons pubis and breast enlargement without secondary contour would be classified on the Tanner Scale as:

    1. Tanner stage I.
    2. Tanner stage II.
    3. Tanner stage III.
    4. Tanner stage IV.

25. A mother of a 2-year-old brings her child to see the nurse practitioner because he has been irritable and has a small "knot" under his left ear. The child has no history of fever, upper respiratory infection, or pulling at his ears. The most likely reason for these symptoms is:

    1. Otitis media.
    2. Teething.

    *hx of irritability + node enlargement lymph node (hx + f) or other symptoms → teething?!*

3. Tonsillitis.
4. Otitis externa.

26. A routine well-child visit for a healthy full-term infant should include a hemoglobin and hematocrit at:

    1. 1 month of age.
    2. 4 months of age.
    3. 6–9 months of age.
    4. 1 year of age.

27. The mother of a 3-month-old infant is concerned because her baby seems to sleep most of the time. The nurse practitioner's response is based on the knowledge that a 3-month-old infant usually spends:

    1. 10 hours in 24 sleeping.
    2. 15–16 hours in 24 sleeping.
    3. 18–19 hours in 24 sleeping.
    4. Most of the 24 hours sleeping, waking only to eat.

28. What advice should the nurse practitioner give a mother who reports during a routine well-child exam that her 5-month-old (weight, 15 lbs), who was sleeping all night at 3 months of age, is now waking up in the middle of the night hungry. A diet history reveals that the infant is taking six 6-ounce bottles of formula in a 24-hour period and has 2 tbsp of rice cereal in the morning.

    1. Increase the amount of formula at each feeding to 8 ounces.
    2. Take the child off formula and switch to homogenized milk.
    3. Decrease the amount of formula to 32 ounces in 24 hours and add fruits, cereals, and juices.   *1-8oz bottle*
    4. Continue the same amount of formula and introduce a variety of baby foods.

29. The father of a 12-year-old male tells the nurse practitioner that he is afraid that his son is getting "fat." The child is at the 50th percentile for height and the 75th percentile for weight on the growth chart. The most appropriate response would be:

    1. Reassure the father that the son is not "fat."

2. Assess family for presence for obesity.

3. Suggest a low-calorie, low-fat diet.

4. Explain that this is typical of the growth pattern of boys at this age.

30. A mother asks the nurse practitioner if an infant walker will help her 6-month-old to learn to walk faster. The nurse practitioner's response is based on the knowledge that:

1. Infant walkers help to strengthen the infant's extremities and prepare them to walk.

2. Infants who are placed in walkers usually walk about 1 month earlier than other infants. *infant walker may delay crawling*

3. Infant walkers are dangerous and should not be recommended for use.

4. There have been very few injuries related to the use of infant mobile walkers.

31. The mother of a 6-month-old infant tells the nurse practitioner that the baby was spitting up his formula so she put him on goat milk. The nurse practitioner is concerned because goat milk places the infant at risk of developing:

1. Rickets. *(lack of Vit D)*

2. Scurvy. *(lack of ascorbic acid)*

3. Folic acid deficiency. → *megaloblastic anemia*

4. Botulism.

32. A 1-year-old reaches for the nurse practitioner's stethoscope with his left hand and the father says, "It looks like he is going to be a lefty just like his old man!" The nurse's response is based on the knowledge that:

1. Male infants usually have the same hand preference as their fathers.

2. Hand preference is well established by 9 months of age.

3. Children will not demonstrate a hand preference until about age 6.

4. Children usually develop handedness by 18–24 months.

*- Children usually develop handedness by 18-24 mos*
*- The hand preference is usually fixed @ 5 years of age*

33. A mother is concerned that her 7-month-old breast-fed infant is not getting enough to eat. The infant weighed 7 lb 8 oz at birth and was 19 inches long. At 6 months of age, he weighed 15 lb and was 25 inches long. He now weighs 15 lb and is 25½ inches long. The nurse practitioner's response is based on the knowledge that:

1. Infants should gain 2–4 oz/wk and ½ inch in height a month during the first six months of life.

2. Infants should triple their birth weight by 6 months of age.  *-0-6 mos | gain 7 oz/d 1"/mo*

3. Infants should gain 3–4 oz/wk and ½ inch in height a month from 6 to 12 months of age.  *-6-12 mo | ½ oz/d ½ in/mo*

4. Infants should gain 1–2 oz/wk and 1 inch in height a month from 6 to 12 months of age.

34. A child will be able to do which of the following fine motor skills first?

1. Imitate a circle. *@ 30 mos*

2. Copy a square. *@ 4 y°*

3. Copy a triangle. *@ 5 y°*

4. Copy a diamond. *@ 6 y°*

35. The nurse practitioner would expect a child to follow a one-step command given without a gesture and using only four to six individual words at what age?

1. 7 months.

2. 9 months.

3. 14 months.

4. 20 months.

36. The nurse practitioner knows that language is the best single measure of normal cognitive development in early childhood. At what age do children begin to combine two words together?

1. 8–10 months.

2. 10–12 months.

3. 12–15 months.

4. 14–23 months.

37. A mother of 2-year-old twins is concerned that the twins do not talk very much and seem to have their own "private" language. The nurse practitioner should:

    1. Tell the mother to spend some individual time with the twins so that they learn language skills.

    2. Perform a pure tone audiometry.

    3. Tell the mother that this is normal for twins or siblings who are close in age.

    4. Refer to a speech pathologist for further testing.

38. The nurse practitioner notices that a 9-month-old infant who was born 2 months prematurely only reaches for an object with his left hand. The nurse would:

    1. Record these findings as normal for a premature infant.

    2. Refer the infant for further evaluation.

    3. Order a muscle biopsy to rule out muscular dystrophy.

    4. Make a note on the chart that the child will probably be left-handed.

39. A mother of a 6-month-old infant tells the nurse practitioner that her infant is now taking homogenized milk instead of an iron-fortified infant formula. The nurse practitioner's response would be based on the knowledge that:

    1. Homogenized milk has the same solute load as formula and is a safe alternative to iron-fortified formula if vitamin supplements are given.

    2. There is an increased incidence of occult gastrointestinal bleeding and the development of iron deficiency anemia in infants fed homogenized milk before 1 year of age.

    3. Once the infant is taking solid foods regularly, there is no need to continue offering iron-fortified formula.

    4. Homogenized milk has too high a fat content and needs to be diluted 2:1 with water.

40. The development of the male sexual characteristics in utero is dependent on:

    1. Estrogen.

    2. Progesterone.

    3. Prolactin.

    4. Testosterone.

41. The production of sperm usually begins during the:

    1. Eighth week of gestation.

    2. Beginning of puberty.

    3. End of puberty.

    4. Eighth month of gestation.

42. What is true about the developmental process of sperm or spermatozoa?

    1. Each mature sperm contain 23 chromosomes.

    2. Sperm become motile immediately at maturation.

    3. Spermatogenesis takes place in the prostate.

    4. Higher than body temperature contributes to sperm production.

43. What do the testes produce?

    1. Alkaline phosphate.

    2. Gonadotropin.

    3. Testosterone only.

    4. Acid phosphate.

44. Which statement is correct concerning healthy sexual developmental tasks?

    1. At 9 years of age, children are less self-conscious and readily expose themselves to younger children or parents of the opposite sex.

    2. At 16 years of age, adolescents are significantly influenced by the media in terms of sexual content and conduct.

    3. At 4 years of age, children distinguish organs associated with each sex and demonstrated increased sexual curiosity.

    4. At 5 years of age, children begin to have concerns about body image and begin to investigate their own sexual organs.

45. The nurse practitioner understands the following about birth defects and growth and development problems in mothers with prenatal alcohol exposure:

    1. If alcohol is ingested late in the pregnancy, there is a higher incidence of postmaturity syndrome.

    2. The practice of drinking alcohol while eating a meal significantly reduces the risk of fully expressed fetal alcohol syndrome.

    3. If alcohol is ingested in large amounts early in the pregnancy, there is an increased incidence of fully expressed clinical features.

    4. Growth retardation is associated with early-trimester alcohol consumption and postmaturity syndrome.

46. In response to a young adult male's question concerning the production of sperm, the nurse practitioner knows that sperm is produced in the:

    1. Epididymis.

    2. Vas deferens.

    3. Prostate.

    4. Seminiferous tubules.

47. An adolescent female with breast budding and sparse, straight, lightly pigmented pubic hair along the medial border of the labia is at which Tanner Stage of Sexual Maturity?

    1. Stage I.

    2. Stage II.

    3. Stage III.

    4. Stage IV.

48. Precocious puberty is defined as:

    1. Onset of puberty before age 8 in females and 9 in males.

    2. Onset of puberty before age 5 in females and 7 in males.

    3. Onset of puberty before age 10 in females and 12 in males.

    4. Onset of puberty for either sex before older siblings enter puberty.

49. The mother of a 5-month-old infant brings her child to the clinic because the infant awakens frequently at night and cries. The nurse practitioner understands that the most common cause of night awakening in healthy infants is:

    1. Night terrors and nightmares.

    2. Separation anxiety.

    3. Trained night crying.

    4. Hunger pain and wet diaper.

50. A 10-day-old breast-fed infant is brought to the clinic because the mother is concerned about the infant's "yellow-orange" color. History and findings are as follows: mother's blood type AB-positive, infant's blood type B-negative, total bilirubin 15 mg/dl. The nurse practitioner understands that this is most likely due to:

    1. Hemolytic jaundice.

    2. Breast-fed jaundice.

    3. Obstructive jaundice.

    4. Physiologic jaundice.

51. A new mother presents to the clinic inquiring about when she should start feeding her 2-month-old infant solid foods. The nurse practitioner should recommend that the mother:

    1. Start the infant on meat and eggs now.

    2. Wait until the infant is 1 year old before introducing solid foods.

    3. Start the infant on cereals now.

    4. Introduce one new food at a time when the infant is 4–6 months old, based on the readiness of the child.

52. All of the following conditions can manifest as failure to thrive in infants except:

    1. Hypothyroidism.

    2. Cystic fibrosis.

    3. Acquired immunodeficiency syndrome (AIDS).

    4. Bronchiolitis.

53. What is considered minimal weight gain in a normal newborn after discharge from the hospital?

    1. 10 gm/day.

    2. 20 gm/day.

    3. 30 gm/day.

    4. 40 gm/day.

54. Which statement is true related to pediatric drug distribution (pharmacokinetics)?

    1. Neonates have an enhanced ability to bind drugs to plasma proteins.

    2. Drug binding reaches adult levels at age 6 years.

    3. Children have a smaller proportion of body fluid for weight; hence there is a lesser volume of distribution or dilution of a drug.

    4. Infants have significantly less ability to bind drugs to plasma proteins due to lower levels of serum albumin, leading to increased risk of toxic effects.

55. The father (74 inches, onset of puberty age 16) of a 15-year-old male adolescent is concerned that his son is going to be short. Upon physical exam, the nurse practitioner finds: Tanner stage II, height 62 inches, physical exam essentially normal for a well-nourished adolescent. After reviewing his growth records, which indicate a growth pattern of height at the 5th percentile, the most likely diagnosis is:

    1. Constitutional growth delay.

    2. Familial short stature.

    3. Hypopituitarism.

    4. Idiopathic gonadotropin deficiency.

# Answers & Rationales

## Physical Assessment

1. **(3)** These are the recommended health evaluation intervals for children to obtain regular assessment information regarding growth and development and to administer recommended immunizations.

2. **(3)** An approach with a well-balanced diet, activity, and exercise are necessary for weight reduction. This allows for slow approach to weight loss that incorporates healthy behavior habits.

3. **(3)** The first and most important part of all data gathering starts with detailed history and physical examination. A detailed, objective description of the dysmorphic features is essential for comparison to textbook descriptions and so forth. Although chromosome analysis will be probably be ordered, it is not done initially. Parents should be included in the discussion of findings and be kept informed of the progress throughout all the evaluation process.

4. **(3)** In-toeing is a common problem and can result from femoral anteversion, adduction of the great toe, medial tibial torsion, and metatarsus adductus. Legg-Calvé-Perthes disease is commonly seen in older children (ages 4–8 years) with loss of hip medial rotation.

5. **(2)** Characteristics of innocent murmurs include midsystolic, asymptomatic, less than a grade III, loudest in pulmonic area (second to third left intercostal space at LSB), no radiation to other areas, may disappear on sitting, and may intensify with fever, activity, anemia, and stress. Any $S_4$ sound is considered pathologic in children as well as adults.

6. **(2)** The posterior fontanel is usually closed by 2 months of age; the anterior closes around 24 months of age.

7. **(3)** Genu varum (bow legs) of 20 degrees is normal up to the age of 18 months.

8. **(1)** Toddlers like to make the first move (i.e., let them move closer and initiate eye contact first; don't call out their name—it may frighten them). Allowing them to handle the stethoscope will decrease their fear. Option #2 is more appropriate when assessing a school-age child.

9. **(2)** Allow a toddler to explore the instruments and start with the extremities. Save the most invasive examination (of the head) for last. In infants, auscultate the heart and lungs while the infant is quiet and then proceed to do a head-to-toe assessment. In the school-age child and adolescent, a head-to-toe sequence is preferred.

10. **(1)** Ishihara's—tests for color perception; Bruchner's—tests for the red reflex; Hirschberg's—tests corneal light reflex; Jaeger's—tests near vision.

11. **(3)** Assessing cranial nerves can be a challenging task for the nurse practitioner; consequently, she should employ techniques that take into consideration the child's developmental level.

12. **(2)** The DDST-R is used for infants through age 5½ years. It is interpreted as normal, suspect, or untestable and measures personal/social areas, fine and gross motor skills, and language. Option #3 is the Denver Articulation Screening Exam (DASE) and Option #4 refers to the age group used for the Early Language Milestone Scale (ELM).

13. **(2)** Genu valgum (knock knee) is considered normal from the age of 2 to the age of 6.

14. **(3)** Mongolian spots are commonly found in African-American, Hispanic, Native American, and Oriental infants. These spots are benign and tend to fade and disappear by age 3, requiring no intervention/treatment. Abuse is not suspected because signs of a healthy mother–infant relationship are noted, namely mother and infant respond positively to one another, and the baby is thriving.

15. **(2)** The plantar fat pad is normal to the age of 2–3 years old.

16. **(2)** Once the tentative diagnosis is made, the nurse practitioner should refer to a pediatric endocrinologist for further work-up. It is beyond the scope of the practitioner's practice to treat at this point.

17. **(2)** Early adolescence is a time when children undergoing great physical changes continually wonder if they are normal. To verbally affirm areas of normalcy during the exam can decrease anxiety.

18. **(2)** Although all areas would be assessed, pregnancy is a common reason for midmorning syncope in adolescents—associated with altered nutrition.

19. **(4)** Newborns and infants up to age 2 months may develop kernicterus as sulfas displace bilirubin from the plasma proteins.

# Growth & Development

20. **(2)** Genetics is the primary determinant of the timing of puberty. Other factors, including geographic location, exposure to light, nutritional status, and health status,

all play a role, but genetics is the major influence.

21. **(4)** Menarche usually occurs about 18–24 months after the onset of breast development. Bone age and labs are not necessary since development is within the normal limits. The findings are not indicative of a chromosomal abnormality; therefore chromosome analysis is unnecessary.

22. **(2)**

| Stage | Pubic Hair |
| --- | --- |
| I | None |
| II | Countable; straight; increased pigmentation and length |
| III | Darker; begins to curl; increased quantity |
| IV | Increased quantity; coarser texture; covers most of pubic area |
| V | Adult distribution; spread to medial thighs and lower abdomen |
| | Genital Development |
| I | Prepubertal |
| II | Testicular enlargement; slight rugation of scrotum |
| III | Further testicular enlargement; penile lengthening begins |
| IV | Testicular enlargement continues; increased rugation of scrotum; increased penile length |
| V | Adult |

23. **(4)** Menarche usually occurs about 18–24 months after the onset of breast development. The average age of menarche is 12.8 years, but that is not what the nurse practitioner should base her response on. Most girls have a growth spurt at Tanner stage IV.

24. **(3)**

| Stage | Pubic Hair |
| --- | --- |
| I | None |
| II | Countable; straight; increased pigmentation and length |
| III | Darker; begins to curl; increased quantity on mons pubis |
| IV | Increased quantity; coarser texture; labia and mons well covered |
| V | Adult distribution, with feminine triangle and spread to medial thighs |

| | Breast Development |
|---|---|
| I | None |
| II | Breast bud present; increased areolar size |
| III | Further enlargement of breast; no secondary contour |
| IV | Areolar area forms secondary mound on breast contour |
| V | Mature; areolar area is part of breast contour; nipple projects |

25. **(2)** At approximately 20 months of age the lower second molars erupt, and at 24 months of age the upper second molars erupt. With a history of irritability and lymph node enlargement without fever or other symptoms, teething is the most likely cause of discomfort.

26. **(3)** It is important in a healthy infant to check the hemoglobin and hematocrit between 6 and 9 months of age when the maternal hemoglobin stores have been depleted. Before 4 months of age, the infant has not depleted his hemoglobin stores. One would not want to wait until 1 year of age to check hemoglobin.

27. **(2)** Normally 3-month-old infants sleep 15–16 hours in a 24-hour period.

28. **(3)** Consumption of 32 oz of formula per day is usually an indicator of the need for solids. Formula is recommended for the first year of life. Nutritional requirements are 110/120 cal/kg/day. Introduction of solids usually occurs between 4 and 6 months of age.

29. **(4)** It is normal for boys at this age to appear heavier before they get their "growth spurt." Reassuring the father, although appropriate, is not the best response. Since the findings are within normal limits, it would not be necessary to assess the family for the presence of obesity. Low-calorie, low-fat diets are contraindicated for the growing child.

30. **(3)** The American Academy of Pediatrics Committee on Injury and Poison Control made a statement recommending a ban on the manufacture and sale of mobile infant walkers. Infant walkers may delay crawling. Up to 35% of infants who use walkers sustain an injury requiring medical attention. Stairs are a very real danger and have caused deaths.

31. **(3)** Goat milk can cause folic acid deficiency, which can lead to megaloblastic anemia. Rickets is caused by the lack of vitamin D. Scurvy is caused by a lack of ascorbic acid in the diet. Botulism is food poisoning caused by an endotoxin produced by the bacillus *Clostridium botulinum.* Most botulism occurs after eating improperly canned or cooked foods. Infants have been known to develop botulism from raw honey that is placed on their pacifiers.

32. **(4)** Children usually develop handedness by 18–24 months. The hand preference is usually fixed after 5 years of age.

33. **(3)** Infants should gain 3–4 oz/wk and ½ inch in height a month from 6 to 12 months of age. This child also doubled its birth weight by 6 months of age as expected.

| | Weight | Length/Height |
|---|---|---|
| 0–6 months | 6–8 oz/wk (doubles birth weight by 5–7 months) | 1 in/mo |
| 6–12 months | 3–4 oz/wk (triples birth weight by 1 year) | ½ in/mo |

34. **(1)** A child should be able to imitate a circle at 30 months; copy a square at 4 years; copy a triangle at 5 years; copy a diamond at 6 years.

35. **(3)** A child should be expected to follow a one-step command given without a gesture and using only four to six individual words between 10.5 and 16.5 months of age.

36. **(4)** Two-word combinations are expected at 14–23 months of age.

37. **(3)** It is normal for twins or sibling close in age to develop a "private" language understood only by them. Although it is important for the mother to spend individual time with each child, this is not what the question is asking. Pure tone audiometry is done after age 3. There is no need for a referral to a speech pathologist at this time.

38. **(2)** The infant should be referred for further evaluation. Handedness before 1 year of age may be an early sign of cerebral palsy. The history of prematurity could be an indication of anoxia at birth and would warrant further investigation. The earlier a child is diagnosed; the earlier intervention can be started.

39. **(2)** Homogenized milk does not have the same solute load as formula and is not a safe alternative to iron-fortified formula even if vitamin supplements are given. The solute load of whole milk is too hard on the infant's immature kidneys. The infant needs to continue taking iron-fortified formula for the first year of life if at all possible. There is an increased incidence of occult gastrointestinal bleeding and the development of iron deficiency anemia in infants fed homogenized milk before 1 year of age.

40. **(4)** The most important sex hormone during embryonic development is the primary male sex hormone, testosterone. Testosterone is produced by the gonads of the genetic male embryo, causing the male gonads to develop into testes, which produce sperm. The other hormones are female hormones. Estrogen, the major female hormone, is produced by the ovaries (ovarian follicle and corpus luteum) and cortices of the adrenal glands and placenta during pregnancy. Progesterone, the second major female hormone, is produced by the corpus luteum. Prolactin is an anterior pituitary hormone and one of the somatotropic hormones that is secreted by lactotropic cells and targets the breast to cause milk production.

41. **(3)** Between the ages of 9 and 12 years the gonads produce more of the sex hormones, which triggers sexual maturation or puberty. Puberty in males begins at approximately age 11 and lasts for 2–3 years, ending with the first ejaculation that contains mature sperm.

42. **(1)** Each mature sperm develops from mitotic division of a diploid (46-chromosome) germ cell (spermatogonium) found on the basement membrane of each seminiferous tubule, which becomes two primary spermatocytes with 23 chromosomes each. Each of these two cells further divides into two more cells (spermatids), with each having 23 chromosomes. Motility is dependent on the biochemicals in semen and in the female reproductive tract. Sperm production needs a temperature that is less than body temperature by at least 1–2 degrees.

43. **(2)** The testes have two functions, the production of gonadotropin (androgens and testosterone) and gametes (sperm). The sperm are produced in the seminiferous tubules of the testes. The androgens and testosterone are produced mainly by Leydig cells of the testes (androgens and testosterone are also produced by the adrenal glands).

44. **(2)** Adolescents are greatly influenced by the media and tend to identify with their parents as sexually functioning people. At age 9, children are more interested in their own body and are quite self-conscious. Option #3 is true for 6-year-olds, not 4-year-olds. Option #4 is true for 10-year-olds.

45. **(3)** Large amounts of alcohol early in the pregnancy have the most devastating effects on the maturing fetus. There is no safe, established dose for alcohol in pregnancy. Food consumption along with alcohol intake does not reduce the risk of defects. Ingesting alcohol in the later months of pregnancy is associated with an increased incidence of premature and small-for-gestational age neonates.

46. **(4)** The sperm are produced in the seminiferous tubules of the testes.

47. **(2)** Tanner has 5 stages of sexual maturity for both males and females; stage I for both is preadolescent and stage V for both is mature or adult development. Stages II, III, and IV chronicle development of breasts, pubic hair distribution, penis, and testis. This young female is demonstrating characteristics of Tanner stage II. (See table in rationale for question 24.)

48. **(1)** Precocious puberty is defined as that which begins at age 8 for females and age 9 for males.

49. **(3)** Trained night crying can become a problem in infants who are not allowed to learn to self-quiet. Activities such as rocking to sleep, exciting play activities before

bedtime, and picking the infant up as soon as he cries can lead to trained night crying. Separation anxiety occurs in infants after 6 months of age. The majority of infants after 4 months of age are able to sleep through the night. Nightmares and night terrors occur at a later age.

50. **(2)** This is a type of exaggerated physiologic jaundice that occurs frequently in breast-fed babies due to the infant's inadequate caloric intake that occurs prior to the mother's milk coming in. It typically occurs between 7 and 15 days of life, whereas physiologic jaundice occurs most commonly after the third day of life. Hemolytic jaundice occurs in an Rh-negative mother who has an Rh-positive infant that becomes isoimmunized.

51. **(4)** Solid foods are not recommended until the infant is 4–6 months old. Cereals should be introduced first, followed by fruits, vegetables, meats, and eggs. All foods should be introduced based on the readiness of the child.

52. **(4)** Many disorders may manifest themselves as organic failure to thrive in children, including congenital heart disease, chronic renal failure, inflammatory bowel disease, chronic liver disease, anorexia, bulimia, and tuberculosis. Nonorganic causes relate to parental neglect, errors in feeding, and maternal deprivation.

53. **(3)** Approximately 30 gm/day is considered adequate weight gain for the newborn. If weight is less than this, the infant may not be thriving.

54. **(4)** Neonates and infants have significantly less ability to bind drugs to plasma proteins due to lower levels of serum albumin, leading to increased risk of toxic effects. Drug binding reaches adult levels at age 6 months to 1 year. Children have a greater proportion of body fluid for weight; hence there is a greater volume of distribution or dilution of a drug.

55. **(1)** Familial short stature is not indicated here as the father is of normal height. Hypopituitarism would be associated with other findings: micropenis, small testes, immature facies, and olfactory defects. Gonadotropin deficiency might be a possibility but, when considering all the findings in the situation and based on the history of the father having a pubertal onset at age 16 and achieving an average height, the more likely diagnosis is constitutional growth delay.

# Health Promotion & Maintenance

1. An adolescent client is continuing his recovery at home after an extensive surgery. The practitioner would instruct the client to increase his intake of what foods to promote healing? *needs ↑ protein + vit C*

   1. Tomatoes, rice, whole bran cereal.

   2. Milk, poultry, yellow vegetables.

   3. Red meat, oranges, green beans.

   4. Liver, corn, eggs.

2. The age group that should be targeted to be taught testicular self-examination would include which ages?

   1. 10–14 years.

   2. 15–25 years.

   3. 30–40 years.

   4. 45–65 years.

3. The recommended number of servings of the bread/cereal/pasta/rice group is how many servings per days?

   1. 6–11 servings.

   2. 2–4 servings.

   3. 3–5 servings.

   4. 2–3 servings.

4. The history collected on a new adolescent client who enters a practice is to include:

   1. Interval history, past medical and surgical history, family medical and surgical histories, immunizations, psychosocial history, usual dietary habits, physical activity, tobacco and other substance use, sexual practices, and a review of systems.

   2. Interval history, past medical history, family medical history, dietary habits, substance use, and sexual practices.

   3. Past medical and surgical histories, family medical history, immunization, psychosocial history, physical activity, tobacco and other substance use, and sexual practices.

   4. The history listed on the form provided to clients for completion prior to the physical examination is sufficient and no interview needs to be done.

5. The most common cause of infant deaths worldwide is:

    1. Pneumonia.

    2. Dehydration.

    3. Acquired immunodeficiency syndrome.

    4. β-Hemolytic streptococcus infections.

6. An appropriate treatment for overweight children under 8 years of age would include:

    1. Administer an appetite suppressant.

    2. Eliminate all carbohydrates in the diet.

    3. Plan a program of activity and exercise.

    4. Use vitamin therapy and herbal teas.

7. When a child comes in for a health maintenance clinic visit, what is essential for the nurse practitioner to do?

    1. Order routine laboratory tests.

    2. Perform vision and auditory screening.

    3. Plot height and weight on charts.

    4. Review immunization record.

8. The nurse practitioner is developing written materials on health care information for parents. Guidelines for developing education materials at an acceptable reading level include all **except**:

    1. Present the most important material first.

    2. Use all capital letters.

    3. Keep sentences short and to the point.

    4. Add visual graphic images to clarify information.

9. In explaining the purpose of primary prevention programs to a group of nursing students, the nurse practitioner relates that primary prevention programs:

    1. Work to lower the incidence of birth defects.

    2. Emphasize early diagnosis and treatment of pediatric anomalies.

    3. Minimize the handicapping effect of mental retardation.

    4. Focus on the prevention of complications and rehabilitation.

10. A healthy 4-month-old infant weighing 13 lb 3 oz has started waking up at night after previously sleeping for 9–11 hours. The infant takes 33 oz of formula in a 24-hour period. The nurse practitioner recommends:

    1. Increase the formula to 38 oz in a 24-hour period.

    2. Start introducing one food item at a time, beginning with vegetables.

    3. Reduce the formula to 28 oz and start small amounts of rice cereal.

    4. Change over to whole milk instead of formula.

11. The nurse practitioner understands that the infant mortality rate is:

    1. The number of infant deaths under 1 year of age per 1000 live births.

    2. The total number of infant deaths per 1000 population.

    3. The number of deaths attributed to specific illnesses.

    4. The monthly newborn death rates per 100 live births.

12. Safety tips for a 6-year-old are:

    1. Wear a life vest when swimming alone.

    2. Teach the child proper use of any guns in the home.

    3. Wear a helmet when bike riding.

    4. Sit in the front seat of the car with seat belt secured.

13. Anticipatory guidance for the family of a 9-month-old includes all **except**:

    1. Use of shoes for protection, not support.

    2. Encourage self-feeding.

    3. Baby-proof home; pool and water safety.

    4. Issues of independence and dependence.

14. The nurse practitioner taking a history on a preschooler learns that the family does not have fluoridated drinking water. Taking into consideration the concerns about fluorosis, the most appropriate nursing intervention would be to:

    1. Prescribe 5 ml of 0.2% fluoride solution rinse (Fluorinse) once daily.

    2. Instruct parents to use a pea-size fluoridated dentifrice and to supervise toothbrushing.

    3. Instruct parents to use bottled drinking water.

    4. Refer to dentist for topical application of fluoride.

15. In teaching a new mother about fevers, the nurse practitioner knows that:

    1. Fevers of 40°C (104°F) can cause brain damage.

    2. All fevers over 40°C (104°F) are usually of bacterial origin.

    3. Children under 6 months of age are especially susceptible to brain damage from a fever.

    4. High fevers may precipitate convulsions in children between 6 months and 6 years of age.

16. A new mother asks about the differences between human milk and cow's milk. The nurse practitioner explains:

    1. Human milk has more antibodies, lipase, and linoleic acid.

    2. Human milk has more calcium, phosphorus, sodium, and potassium.

    3. Cow's milk has low protein and casein content.

    4. Cow's milk has high linoleic acid and low saturated fatty acids.

17. The nurse practitioner recognizes the following as correct for the frequency and quantity of formula feedings:

    1. 1 month: 9–10 feedings/24 hours of 2–3 oz.

    2. 6 months: 8–10 feedings/24 hours of 4–5 oz.

    3. 10 months: 4–5 feedings/24 hours of 7–8 oz.

    4. 12 months: 6–8 feedings/24 hours of 8–9 oz.

18. According to the American Academy of Pediatrics (AAP), infants may be fed whole cow's milk once they reach:

    1. 6 months of age.

    2. 8 months of age.

    3. 12 months of age.

    4. 18 months of age.

19. A mother states that the iron-fortified formula her 3-month-old infant is on has been causing constipation. The nurse practitioner recommends:

    1. Discontinuing the iron-fortified formula.

    2. Starting the infant on rice cereal.

    3. Adding 1–2 tsp of dark corn syrup to formula.

    4. Avoiding prune, apricot, and pineapple juices.

20. Which of the following describes lactose intolerance?

    1. Children usually exhibit symptoms around 4–6 years of age. Symptoms typically include intestinal dilatation, bloating, increased flatulence, and pain followed eventually by diarrhea.

    2. Infants and toddlers are typically affected. Symptoms occur within 30 minutes after eating milk products or drinking milk and are characterized by abrupt onset of nausea, vomiting, and diarrhea.

    3. It is the same as cow's milk intolerance.

    4. Its prevalence is highest among the Caucasian population.

21. A routine lab study is returned to the nurse practitioner on a 1-year-old who had a normal yearly exam. The lead level is reported as 15 µg/dl. The nurse practitioner takes which action?

    1. Repeat the test since it may be a false result.

    2. Hospitalize for immediate chelation therapy.

    3. Investigate possible sources of lead and repeat in 6 months.

    4. Repeat the test in 1 year.

22. The recommended time for introduction of solid foods into an infant's diet is:

    1. Age 2 months.

    2. Age 4–6 months.

    3. Age 6–8 months.

    4. Age 3 months.

23. The nurse practitioner is aware that fluoride levels in drinking water should be:

    1. 0.5 ppm in temperate and cold climates.

    2. 1.0 ppm in temperate and 0.5 ppm in cold climates.

    3. 1.0 ppm in temperate and cold climates.

    4. 0.6 ppm in temperate and 1.0 ppm in cold climates.

24. A 20-day-old infant is brought to the clinic by her parents. She has not been eating well and has a temperature of 38.2°C (100.8°F). Upon exam, no focal bacterial infection is found, lab indicates a white blood cell (WBC) count of 12,000/mm³ with 1480 bands/mm³, urinalysis is normal, and there is no diarrhea noted. Management involves:

    1. Treat at home with antipyretics and fluids.

    2. Hospitalize for a septic work-up.

    3. Treat at home with antipyretics and ampicillin.

    4. Do a urine culture and have the infant return in 24 hours.

25. In teaching the fifth- through eighth-grade child about health promotion behaviors, it is important to remember that:

    1. Girls are more extrinsically motivated.

    2. Both boys and girls are highly influenced by family.

    3. Boys are more extrinsically motivated.

    4. High maternal education levels affect both.

26. In the preparation of reading and education materials for clients and parents, the nurse practitioner is aware that the reading level of most adults is at the:

    1. 12th grade level.

    2. 10th grade level.

    3. 6th grade level.

    4. 4th grade level.

27. A child presenting with vague symptoms and a serum lead level of 28 µg/dl would be managed by:

    1. Removal of the child from the lead source.

    2. Removal of the environmental lead hazard.

    3. Chelation therapy treatment.

    4. Rescreen and referral to physician.

28. Primary injury prevention teaching for the parents of a 2-month-old includes:

    1. Set water heater thermostat at <120°F.

    2. Make sure crib rails are no more than 3¾ inches apart.

    3. Use a rear-facing car seat until the child is >40 lb.

    4. Apply sunscreen when outside and temperature is above 75°F.

29. Discussion of home/folk remedies utilized by the Hispanic family of a child with vague symptoms of weakness, irritability, weight loss, constipation, and mild ataxia and a previous history of elevated lead levels might reveal the use of:

    1. White willow bark.

2. Arnica root.

3. Mexican yam root.

4. Azarcon and greta.

30. Anticipatory guidance for the parents of a 26-week-gestation premature infant who is going home after 2 months in the neonatal intensive care unit (NICU) would include the infant's need for:

    1. Fluoride supplement due to lack of breast feeding.

    2. Lights to be on 24 hours a day.

    3. Decreased handling and stimulation.

    4. Bright colors and continuous music for stimulation.

31. A new mother has weaned her 2-month-old and started her on formula. During the past week, the mother has noted that the infant's stools are becoming constipated and she is having only one or two hard bowel movements per week. The infant's physical exam reveals soft, nontender abdomen; vital signs normal; and several light brown, hard stools in the diaper. What would the nurse practitioner do?

    1. Tell the mother to give the infant a glycerin suppository and use it bid for 2 weeks.

    2. Explain that this is normal and the infant will usually have a constipated stool until food is introduced.

    3. Write a prescription for 10–15 ml of milk of magnesia at HS, prn.

    4. Encourage the mother to offer more fluids, including prune juice.

32. An infant is in for a 2-month well-baby check. Weight at birth was 4 lb 2 oz, at 1 month was 5 lb 6 oz, and 2 months is 6 lb 6 oz. What is appropriate teaching to give to a new mother who tells the nurse practitioner that her infant "spits up" after taking her bottle?

    1. Have the mother burp the infant more often throughout the feeding.

    2. Refer the infant to the pediatrician for a pyloric stenosis work-up.

3. Have the mother reduce the amount of formula at each feeding by 10 ml.

4. Explain to the mother that the infant will grow out of the "spitting up" phase.

33. What are the recommendations of the Centers for Disease Control (CDC) for screening for lead poisoning?

    1. No specific guidelines recommended.

    2. Annually, starting at age 1 year.

    3. Between 6 months and 6 years of age.

    4. Every other year starting at age 1.

# Immunizations

34. The mother of a 2-month-old refuses to have her child vaccinated with the trivalent oral polio vaccine (OPV) because she has read that some children can get polio from the vaccine. The nurse practitioner's best action would be:

    1. Respect the mother's choice, do not give the vaccine.

    2. Explain the seriousness of polio if the child does not get the vaccine.

    3. Discuss the three different acceptable schedules for polio vaccination.

    4. Give the vaccine as it is a state law and is required on all infants.

35. Before giving a child the measles-mumps-rubella (MMR) trivalent vaccine, it is recommended to wait how long after cancer chemotherapy has stopped?

    1. 30 days.

    2. 2 months.

    3. 3 months.

    4. 6 months.

36. The National Childhood Vaccine Injury Act requires standardized consent forms for the administration of vaccines to children. The content on the form for the medical record includes the vaccine lot number, nurse signature, injection/inoculation site, and:

    1. Parental signature.

    2. Education provided.

    3. Absence of contraindications.

    4. Vaccine expiration date.

37. The mother of a 15-year-old who has not had chickenpox is concerned and wants her daughter to be vaccinated. The recommendations are:

    1. Not recommended for children over age 12.

    2. A one-time dose.

    3. Three doses 2 months apart.

    4. Two doses 4–8 weeks apart.

38. Consultation with the mother of an 18-month-old who has received no immunizations reveals that the child was exposed to measles 48 hours prior to the visit. At this time the practitioner would:

    1. Discharge the client with care instructions.

    2. Administer live attenuated measles vaccine.

    3. Administer 0.5 ml/kg immunoglobulin G (IgG).

    4. Administer half the regular measles vaccine dose.

39. The nurse practitioner understands that the only contraindication to hepatitis B vaccination is:

    1. Pregnancy and lactation.

    2. History of poliomyelitis.

    3. Prior anaphylaxis or severe hypersensitivity.

    4. Mild viral illness.

40. The nurse practitioner understands that the following is considered an attenuated live-virus vaccination:

    1. Rubella and measles.

    2. Mumps and hepatitis B.

    3. Poliomyelitis and hepatitis B.

    4. Rubella and rabies.

41. The nurse practitioner understands that children who are at high risk of an adverse reaction to the measles vaccine are children who have severe allergic reactions to:

    1. Fungi.

    2. Pollen.

    3. Pets.

    4. Food.

42. What type of immunity does a child develop after he has contracted chickenpox?

    1. Actively acquired immunity.

    2. Artificially acquired immunity.

    3. Natural passive immunity.

    4. Naturally acquired active immunity.

43. The nurse practitioner is assessing an 8-month-old infant in an immunization clinic. The nurse practitioner knows that by 8 months the child should have had which immunizations?

    1. Hepatitis B (Hep B) first and second does, all of the primary diphtheria-tetanus-pertussis (DTaP) series, and two doses of the polio series.

    2. All of the DTaP and polio series, MMR.

    3. DTaP first and second dose, MMR first dose, all of the Hep B series.

    4. Varicella, DTaP first dose, Hep B first dose.

44. In considering client situations, which one requires the use of an inactivated (not live) vaccine?

    1. History of nonspecific allergies.

    2. Immunocompromised client.

    3. Concurrent antimicrobial therapy.

    4. Mild acute illness.

45. Immunizations recommended for a healthy 19-year-old include:

    1. Measles, rubella, varicella, and hepatitis B.

    2. Pneumovax, influenza, and rubella.

    3. Tetanus, influenza, varicella, Pneumovax, and hepatitis B.

    4. Influenza, hepatitis B, rubella, measles, tetanus, and varicella.

46. A 2-month-old infant received his immunizations and 12 hours later the mother calls and says that the infant has a fever of 101°F. What is the most likely cause of the fever?

    1. The vaccination for the measles, mumps, and rubella.

    2. The combination of the diphtheria and the polio vaccinations.

    3. The presence of an infection when immunizations were given.

    4. The pertussis immunization.

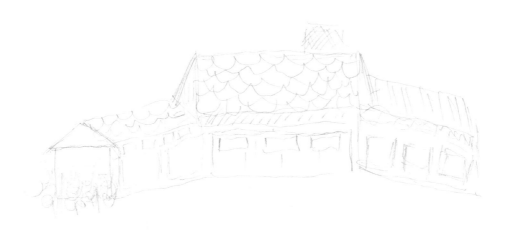

3 - Hep
4 - Hib, IPV
5 - Dtap

* immunizations
@ 2mos — hEp¹, Hib¹ Dtap¹, IPV¹, Prev¹
@ 4mos — hep 2, Hib² Dtap², IPV², Prev²
@ 6mos — hep 3, Hib³ Dtap³, IPV³, Prev³
@ 9mos — Catchup
@ 1Yr-15mos — MMR¹, Varicella, Hib⁴, Pre⁴
@ 15-18mos — Dtap⁴
@ 2Y° = HepA¹
2.6Y° = HepA²
@ 4Y° — MMR², Dtap⁵, IPV⁴
@ 11Y° = Dt

# Answers & Rationales

1. **(3)** The client needs an increased intake of protein and vitamin C to promote healing. Red meat, citrus fruits, and green vegetables will give the highest amounts of these elements from the selections offered.

2. **(2)** The 15–25 age group is most commonly affected by testicular cancer.

3. **(1)** The recommended servings for each of the food groups are as follows:

| Food Group | Servings |
| --- | --- |
| Bread/cereal/rice/pasta | 6–11 servings |
| Fruit group | 2–4 servings |
| Vegetable group | 3–5 servings |
| Meat/poultry/fish, dry beans, eggs & nuts group | 2–3 servings |
| Fats/oils/sweets | Sparing uses |

4. **(1)** All of these areas are important to probe in the initial interview of a new adolescent client. The history will help determine the necessary components of the physical examination and laboratory or radiologic studies that are ordered and the counseling that is done during the appointment.

5. **(2)** Dehydration results in the deaths of more infants worldwide than any other syndrome.

6. **(3)** An approach with a well-balanced diet, activity, and exercise are necessary for weight reduction. This allows for a slow approach to weight loss that incorporates healthy behavior habits.

7. **(4)** It is absolutely essential that the immunization record be reviewed. The other options are important but are not essential for a health maintenance visit.

8. **(2)** Printed materials must be written at a level of readability at which they can be understood. Do not use all capital letters, as words so written are difficult to read. Also, it is helpful to write in the active versus the passive voice, to use one- and two-syllable words, to avoid complex grammatical structures, and to express only one idea in each sentence.

9. **(1)** Primary prevention programs exist to prevent disease, malfunctioning, or maladaptation from occurring. Examples of these types of programs include promoting a healthy diet, practicing safe sex, and avoiding alcohol and tobacco use. Secondary prevention is early diagnosis and treatment (i.e., screening for tuberculosis or sickle cell disease, breast and testicular self-examination). Tertiary prevention is the prevention of complications and rehabilitation after the disease or condition has already occurred (i.e., cardiac rehabilitation, having a complete blood count [CBC] drawn before chemotherapy).

10. **(3)** If the infant has been satisfied up to this point (by sleeping for long intervals), more than likely he needs additional calories in the form of rice cereal. Adding increased amounts of formula can lead to iron deficiency anemia.

11. **(1)** This is a commonly used ratio that is calculated as follows:

$$\frac{\text{No. of deaths} < 1 \text{ year of age in a year}}{\text{No. of live births in the same year}}$$
$$\times\ 1000 = \text{Infant mortality rate}$$

12. **(3)** Bike safety includes wearing a helmet; stopping at a curb; looking left, then right, then left again, before crossing a street; and no riding in the street until older. Children should always wear life vests, but should not swim alone. Although firearm safety is important, a 6-year-old is too young to learn to handle a firearm. It is best to keep all firearms out of the home; if kept in the home, keep them unloaded and locked in a place separate from ammunition. The child should sit in the back seat, as the air bag deployment may injure a child who is sitting in the front seat.

13. **(4)** Issues of independence and dependence are usually discussed with the parents of a 2-year-old. All of the other options are appropriate for anticipatory guidance, along with talking to the child and avoiding bottle tooth decay (no bottle in the bed).

14. **(2)** A fluoridated dentifrice should be used in a small amount (pea-size) and children under 6 should be supervised so that they do not swallow too much toothpaste, which would put them at risk for fluorosis. The dose of fluoride rinse is too high, plus it is inappropriate to prescribe to a preschooler. Bottled water does not contain fluoride. Topical application, though appropriate, is not the best answer.

15. **(4)** Febrile seizures are benign and do not lead to brain damage. Most febrile illness in children is due to a virus rather than a bacteria, and is associated with a high fever.

16. **(1)** Cow's milk is not as good a nutritional source as human milk because it has more mineral content (calcium, potassium, sodium, phosphorus), which causes a larger renal solute load. In addition, cow's milk is high in protein, casein, and saturated fat and lower in carbohydrates, while human milk is rich in antibodies.

17. **(3)** Usual frequency and quantity of formula feedings are as follows:

    0–1 month: 6–8 feedings/24 hours of 2–4 oz.
    2 months: 4–5 feedings/24 hours of 5 oz.
    3 months: 4–5 feedings/24 hours of 5–6 oz.

    4 months: 4–5 feedings/24 hours of 6–7 oz.
    7–10 months: 3–4 feedings/24 hours of 8 oz.
    11–12 months: 3 feedings/24 hours of 8 oz.

18. **(3)** At 1 year of age, infants may be fed whole cow's milk. The purpose for waiting is that it has been shown that cow's milk is low in iron, linoleic acid, and vitamin E, as well as being high in protein, sodium, and potassium.

19. **(3)** The AAP does not recommend low-iron formulas and, if stools are hard, recommends treatment for constipation. Typical treatment includes giving 1–2 tsp of dark corn syrup; including fruit juices (prune, pineapple, apricot), nonstarchy vegetables, water, and avoiding rice cereal.

20. **(1)** These are characteristics of lactose intolerance. Symptoms occur from 2 to as many as 12 hours after milk or milk product ingestion. The prevalence is highest in African-Americans, Native Americans, and Asians. Cow's milk intolerance occurs in infancy and has symptoms of blood in the stools often accompanied by allergies, such as eczema, hives, or asthma.

21. **(3)** While 15 μg/dl is an elevated count (normal level is <10 μg/dl), chelation therapy in children with a normal exam is not usually conducted until the level is >25 μg/dl. It is important at this level to identify the source of the elevation and monitor the child frequently.

22. **(2)** Solid food does not need to be introduced before 4–6 months of age. The first foods introduced are cereals. New foods are introduced one at a time at weekly intervals. In this way, the infant's digestive system can get used to the food and any reaction can be easily detected. Remember to look for a range (i.e., a beginning and ending date) for recommendations.

23. **(4)** Levels recommended by the dental association of 0.6 ppm in temperate climates and 1.0 ppm in cold climates are based on the rationale that people in temperate climates drink more fluids. Intake is determined at 1 L/day. Below this level, children need supplements and they cannot be prescribed without knowing the exact fluoride concentration in the water.

24. **(2)** Practice guidelines recommend that febrile infants under 28 days, even if they meet low risk criteria, should have a sepsis evaluation.

25. **(1)** Fifth- through eighth-grade girls are more motivated by peers and family. Boys are more intrinsically motivated, with family and peers having less influence. Peers are also more influential for girls in the high school years. High maternal education level is not an influential factor for boys.

26. **(3)** The reading level of most American adults is at the sixth grade level.

27. **(4)** The CDC's recommendations for a serum lead level >10 μg/dl are for rescreening and referral to a physician. Rescreening is done prior to removal of the child/family from the hazard, although a thorough environmental assessment is essential at the time of rescreening.

28. **(1)** The water heater should not be set over 120°F to prevent scald burns. Crib rails should be no more than 2⅜ inches apart; the rear-facing infant seat is applicable to 20 pounds and 12 months of age. Sunscreen should be applied whenever there is sun exposure.

29. **(4)** Azarcon and greta are traditional Hispanic remedies that contain lead, which can lead to increased lead levels and eventual poisoning. The other remedies will not cause the symptoms described. The Mexican yam root is utilized for menopausal symptoms and is a source of natural progesterone.

30. **(2)** Premature infants who have spent an extended period of time in the NICU take 6–10 months to be deinstitutionalized to the noise and light. These must be decreased slowly over a period of time.

31. **(4)** Fluids and prune juice are helpful in treating constipation. This is a common problem for formula-fed infants, especially when they have been changed from breast feeding. The constipation is usually due to inadequate fluid intake, a diet too high in fat or protein (which may occur with formula-fed infants), or a diet lacking in bulk. The glycerin suppository and milk of magnesia could be prescribed for temporary relief, but are not recommended as an appropriate measure to deal with the constipation.

32. **(1)** Spitting up, or regurgitation, is a common problem in the infant due to an immature gastroesophageal sphincter. In the absence of poor weight gain or projectile vomiting (which may indicate pyloric stenosis), the infant needs to be burped more frequently throughout the feeding.

33. **(3)** Remember to look for a range (i.e., a beginning and ending date) for recommendations. The CDC recommends screening all children between 6 months and 6 years of age. If a child is developmentally disabled or there is a positive recent or past history, children 6–16 years of age should be screened. Children at highest risk are those of lower socioeconomic status who live in older dwellings and who are 6 months to 6 years of age, with the peak incidence occurring in spring and summer months.

## Immunizations

34. **(3)** It is important for the nurse practitioner to discuss all three options (all OPV; all eIPV, and eIPV-OPV) before obtaining consent from the parent. e-IPV (inactivated trivalent polio vaccine–enhanced) has been proven to be effective against wild polio and is recommended for use by some health experts. The e-IPV can be used for all three doses or in combination with OPV. Therefore, individuals refusing OPV can receive e-IPV.

35. **(3)** The MMR is a live-virus vaccine, and children severely immunosuppressed due to cancer therapy should wait until immunoglobulin levels have increased or they will be at increased risk for serious complications and the disease.

36. **(1)** The law calls for the parental signature to be maintained in the clinical record.

37. **(4)** Children over the age of 13 who have not had chickenpox and have not been previously immunized are recommended to

have two doses 4–8 weeks apart for effective immunity.

38. **(2)** The live attenuated measles vaccine, if given within 72 hours of exposure, will provide protection in most cases. The dose of IgG would be 0.25 ml/kg given within 6 days of exposure.

39. **(3)** Prior anaphylaxis and severe hypersensitivity would be considered a contraindication; a mild viral illness would not. The client who is pregnant or lactating may be immunized.

40. **(1)** Attenuated live-virus vaccines are available for the following communicable diseases: measles, mumps, rubella, poliomyelitis, yellow fever, and smallpox. Rabies vaccine is a killed virus and hepatitis B is a purified viral antigen obtained from the blood of an infected client and then inactivated when manufactured into a vaccine.

41. **(4)** Atopic (allergic) children who have severe food allergy are at an increased risk for the development of an allergic reaction to the measles vaccine. Children with food allergy should be observed for at least 90 minutes in a setting equipped for emergency medical treatment.

42. **(4)** A child who contracts chickenpox for the first time develops antibodies during the period of infection. These antibodies create a naturally acquired, lifelong type of active immunity. Artificially acquired immunity occurs with immunizations. Natural passive immunity occurs with placental transfer.

Active acquired immunity occurs with an injection of human or animal serum.

43. **(1)** Standard immunizations are two doses of Hep B series, all of the initial DTaP series, and two of the polio series. MMR and varicella are not given until 12–15 months.

44. **(2)** Live vaccine can produce serious disseminated disease in a client with an immunocompromising illness such as leukemia, lymphoma, or human immunodeficiency virus/acquired immunodeficiency syndrome (HIV/AIDS) or in clients undergoing cancer chemotherapy. Mild acute illness, concurrent antimicrobial therapy, and a history of nonspecific allergies are not contraindications for use of a live vaccine.

45. **(4)** Five to 20% of young adults are susceptible to measles and/or rubella. Influenza and hepatitis B immunizations are recommended for students who have exposure to a large number of people. Varicella is recommended for susceptible persons. Tetanus is recommended every 10 years, especially in high-risk situations (young adults who participate in outdoor sports). Pneumovax is indicated in a young adult who has a chronic disease, such as diabetes, chronic pulmonary disease, or chronic cardiovascular disease; it is also indicated for young adults who are immunocompromised.

46. **(4)** The most likely cause of fever at the 2-month immunization series is the pertussis. This vaccine causes reactions in about 75% of infants. MMR is not given until 12–15 months of age.

# 4 Cardiovascular

## Physical Examination & Diagnostic Tests

1. The nurse practitioner is performing a physical examination on a healthy child. On auscultation the stethoscope would be placed in what areas to best hear the characteristic sounds of $S_1$ and $S_2$?

   1. $S_1$ is best heard at the apex and $S_2$ at the base of the heart.

   2. Both are heard equally well on the right side at the midclavicular line.

   3. On the left side, $S_1$ is at the area of the pulmonic valve and $S_2$ at the aortic valve.

   4. Both are best heard at Erb's point at the third intercostal space at the sternal margin.

2. On the general assessment of an adolescent client, the practitioner determines the presence of the apical impulse at the point of maximal impulse (PMI) on the client's chest wall. Where on the chest wall is the PMI normally found?

   1. Second intercostal space at the midclavicular line on the left side.

   2. Right lower sternal border, fifth intercostal space.

   3. Left side at the fifth intercostal space on the midclavicular line.

   4. Left fifth intercostal space, lateral to the midclavicular line.

3. When inspecting the precordium, the nurse practitioner is checking for:

   1. Scars and anatomic landmarks.

   2. Pulsations and retractions.

   3. Heaves and cardiac dullness.

   4. Pericardial friction rub and lifts.

4. While examining an adolescent in a left lateral decubitus position, the nurse practitioner auscultates a third heart sound ($S_3$). The nurse practitioner knows:

   1. This sound is normally heard in children and young adults and is considered a physiologic $S_3$.
   2. This rarely is associated with myocardial failure in the adolescent.
   3. This client should be immediately referred to a cardiologist for evaluation.
   4. This is considered a normal splitting of the $S_2$ during inspiration and is accentuated by positioning.

5. The nurse practitioner is examining an older child with a history of rheumatic fever who is being followed for the development of carditis. During the cardiac auscultation, where on the chest wall is the stethoscope placed to determine the most common murmurs associated with this condition?

   1. At the left sternal border, fourth left intercostal space. _Tricuspid valve_
   2. Fifth intercostal space on the left side at the midclavicular line. _Mitral valve_
   3. Second or third intercostal space at the left of the sternal border. _Pulmonic valve_
   4. Second intercostal space on the right of the sternal border. _Aortic valve_

6. $S_1$ and $S_2$ are identified when the nurse practitioner auscultates for cardiac sounds. The physiology responsible for the production of these heart sounds is:

   1. Contraction of the ventricles and closure of the atrioventricular (AV) valves produces $S_1$; closure of the semilunar valves forms $S_2$.
   2. Closure of the aortic valve produces $S_2$; opening of the mitral valve and filling of the left ventricle forms $S_1$.
   3. The opening of the AV valves produces $S_1$; closure of the semilunar valves produces $S_2$.
   4. Opening of the tricuspid produces $S_1$; closure of the pulmonic forms $S_2$.

7. The nurse practitioner notes a grade V systolic murmur while examining a client's

precordium. Which characteristics describe this type of murmur?

   1. Barely audible, faint with the bell of the stethoscope.
   2. Heard only with the diaphragm of the stethoscope.
   3. Heard with the stethoscope partly off the chest.
   4. Heard without the aid of the stethoscope.

8. Upon examination of a child, the nurse practitioner notes weak femoral pulses. This finding is indicative of:

   1. Patent ductus arteriosus.
   2. Coarctation of the aorta.
   3. Tetralogy of Fallot.
   4. Pulmonary stenosis.

9. In doing a cardiac assessment of a 4-month-old infant, the nurse practitioner notes a machinery-like murmur. This finding is consistent with a diagnosis of:

   1. Coarctation of the aorta.
   2. Patent ductus arteriosus.
   3. Ventricular septal defect.
   4. Aortic stenosis.

10. The practitioner is examining an adolescent with a known history of mitral valve disease. What type of murmur heard on auscultation supports a history of mitral stenosis?

    1. Diastolic murmur, heard loudest at the apex with the client on her left side.
    2. Midsystolic ejection murmur, heard loudest over the left lower sternal border. _aortic sten_
    3. Holosystolic murmur, heard loudest over the apex and left axillary area. _mitral regurg_
    4. Diastolic murmur, heard loudest with client in sitting position leaning forward. _aortic regurg_

# Disorders

11. The diagnosis of hypertension (HTN) in an 18-year-old should be established on the basis of:

1. At least three readings with an average systolic blood pressure (BP) of 140 mm Hg and diastolic pressure of 90 mm Hg.

2. At least 5 readings 1 month apart.

3. One reading of 140 mm Hg systolic and 90 mm Hg diastolic or above.

4. One reading taken in three different positions.

12. Two clinical presentations of children with congenital heart disease are symptoms of congestive heart failure (CHF) and:

    1. Hypoglycemia.

    2. Hypertension.

    3. Peripheral edema.

    4. Cyanosis.

13. From the following description, what data most clearly describes atrial tachycardia in an older adolescent?

    1. Heart rate of 96, P waves present on each QRS complex, T wave every other beat.

    2. P waves present on every other beat, heart rate of 100, and irregular.

    3. Heart rate of 120, P waves present prior to each QRS complex, and regular.

    4. P waves for every third QRS complex, adequate P-R interval, heart rate of 90.

14. The nurse practitioner is performing an assessment on a child with left-sided congestive heart failure. The nurse practitioner understands that the primary symptoms associated with this type of failure are:

    1. Systemic venous congestion.

    2. Dyspnea and pulmonary congestion.

    3. Increased peripheral edema and anorexia.

    4. Atrial fibrillation with a heart rate around 110.

15. In evaluating the effectiveness of cardiopulmonary resuscitation (CPR) on the child, the nurse practitioner would note:

    1. Dilated pupils.

    2. Palpable carotid pulse.

    3. Capillary refill within 2 seconds.

    4. Pink and warm skin.

16. When cardiac output falls in congestive heart failure, the body attempts to compensate. What electrolye imbalances occur as a result of this response?

    1. Hypernatremia and hyperkalemia.

    2. Hyponatremia and hypokalemia.

    3. Hypophosphatemia and hypercalcemia.

    4. Hyperphosphatemia and hypocalcemia.

17. Clinical manifestations of congestive heart failure (CHF) in an infant are:

    1. Easily fatigued, central cyanosis, tachycardia, tachypnea, splenomegaly.

    2. Coughing, diaphoresis, peripheral edema, hepatomegaly.

    3. Tachycardia, tachypnea, easily fatigued, paleness, hepatomegaly.

    4. Peripheral edema, coughing, splenomegaly, hepatomegaly, tachycardia.

18. The most common causes of chest pain in children are:

    1. Ischemic heart disease; congestive heart failure (CHF).

    2. Gastroesophageal reflux disease; congenital heart disease (CHD).

    3. Mitral valve prolapse; musculoskeletal.

    4. Idiopathic; musculoskeletal.

19. A young child is scheduled for surgical repair of tetralogy of Fallot. What does the nurse practitioner expect the child's hemoglobin (Hgb) values to show, and what kind of lesion does the child have?

    1. Hgb 18 gm/dl, cyanotic.

    2. Hgb 3 gm/dl, cyanotic.

    3. Hgb 10 gm/dl, acyanotic.

    4. Hgb 18 gm/dl, acyanotic.

20. The nurse practitioner understands that the most likely cause of hypertension in a young child is:

    1. Glomerulonephritis.

    2. Pheochromocytoma.

    3. Rheumatic fever.

    4. Hyperthyroidism.

21. Which of the following would be pertinent on the past medical history of a child who is being evaluated for cardiovascular disease?

    1. Kawasaki's disease.

    2. Hypothyroidism.

    3. Osteogenic sarcoma.

    4. Tourette's syndrome.

22. The nurse practitioner would refer to a pediatric cardiologist for work-up and evaluation within 1–2 weeks a child with:

    1. Signs of exercise intolerance, dyspnea, and elevated pulse.

    2. Poor feeding, increased cyanosis with crying, and dizziness.

    3. Nonfunctional heart murmur, respiratory crackles, and retarded growth and development.

    4. Systolic ejection murmur, grade II, that disappears on sitting.

23. Infective endocarditis prophylaxis may be required for children with congenital heart defects in which of the following conditions?

    1. Dental procedures such as simple adjustment of orthodontic appliances.

    2. Cardiac catheterization.

    3. Tonsillectomy and/or adenoidectomy.

    4. Insertion of tympanostomy tubes.

24. For the child with congenital heart disease (CHD) and a permanent pacemaker, electrical safety precautions include avoidance of:

    1. Cellular phones.

    2. Microwave ovens.

    3. Household electrical appliances.

    4. Metal detectors.

25. A child is being worked up for rheumatic fever. His physical findings are 103.6°F temperature, migratory joint pain, and elevated erythrocyte sedimentation rate (ESR). According to the Jones criteria, what other finding is essential for the diagnosis of rheumatic fever?

    1. History of group A streptococcal throat infection.

    2. Carditis.

    3. Sydenham's chorea.

    4. History of erythema marginatum for past 3 days.

26. The nurse practitioner understands that hypoplastic left heart syndrome is characterized by:

    1. Development of heart failure in the first few weeks of life.

    2. Bounding peripheral pulses.

    3. Absence of dyspnea in spite of circumoral cyanosis.

    4. No hepatomegaly or splenomegaly.

27. Management of a child with hypertension includes:

    1. Strict adherence to avoiding all forms of isometric and regular exercise.

    2. Weight reduction, exercise, moderate salt restriction, and avoidance of tobacco.

    3. Immediately starting the child on an angiotension-converting enzyme (ACE) inhibitor and thiazide diurectic.

    4. Aggressive use of a STEP approach, starting with a vasodilator such as hydralazine (Apresoline).

# Pharmacology

28. An adolescent is started on spironolactone (Aldactone) 50 mg PO qd. The nurse

practitioner instructs the adolescent to call the clinic if which symptoms are experienced?

1. Muscle weakness, fatigue, and nausea.

2. Decreased reflex response, nausea, and vomiting.

3. Muscle twitching, numbness of the limbs, and depression.

4. Weight gain, excessive thirst, and fever.

29. Secondary prophylaxis for acute rheumatic fever (ARF) in an older adolescent includes:

    1. Penicillin V 125–250 mg PO bid indefinitely.

    2. Erythromycin 800 mg PO bid.

3. One-time dose of 2.0 million units benzathine penicillin G combined with penicillin G procaine (Bicillin C-R) IM.

4. No medication prophylaxis is needed after client reaches early 20s.

30. A toddler has ingested some of his grandfather's pills. The toddler is vomiting, feels weak, and has a first-degree AV block pattern on the electrocardiogram. The grandfather brings in four medication bottles. Which is the most likely medication the toddler ingested?

    1. Amitriptyline (Elavil).

    2. Digoxin (Lanoxin).

    3. Furosemide (Lasix).

    4. Aspirin.

# 4 Answers & Rationales

## Physical Examination & Diagnostic Tests

1. **(1)** S$_1$ is heard loudest at the apex, S$_2$ at the base. Each sound should be carefully assessed as to the intensity of the sound in each area.

2. **(3)** The PMI represents the thrust and contraction of the left ventricle (LV). The LV lies behind the right ventricle (RV) and extends to the left, forming the left border of the heart.

3. **(2)** The purpose of inspection and palpation of the precordium is to determine the presence and extent of normal and abnormal pulsations. A slight retraction of the chest wall just medial to the midclavicular line in the fifth interspace is a normal finding, whereas marked or active retraction of the rib is abnormal and may indicate pericardial disease. Pericardial friction rubs are heard by auscultation.

4. **(1)** The splitting during inspiration refers to S$_1$ and S$_2$. The S$_3$ is normal in children, young adults, and pregnant women. In the older adult with heart disease, this often signifies myocardial failure.

5. **(2)** The fifth intercostal space at the midclavicular line on the left side is the best place to auscultate the closure sounds of the mitral valve. Option #1 describes the area of the tricuspid valve. Option #3 describes the area of the pulmonic valve. Option #4 describes the aortic valve area.

6. **(1)** Closure of the AV valves, which allows the filling of both ventricles simultaneously, produces the first heart sound (S$_1$). Closure of the aortic and pulmonic valves produce the second heart sound (S$_2$).

7. **(3)** A grade V heart murmur is very loud and can be heard with the stethoscope partly off the chest wall. A grade VI murmur is the loudest and is audible with the stethoscope just removed from contact with the chest wall and accompanied by a thrill. A grade I is barely audible or very faint with the bell of the stethoscope.

8. **(2)** Weak or absent pulses are associated with coarctation of the aorta and are not indicative of the other cardiovascular diseases listed.

9. **(2)** A machinery-type murmur is consistent with patent ductus arteriosus (PDA). The turbulent flow of blood from the aorta through the PDA to the pulmonary artery results in a characteristic machinery-like murmur. Coarctation presents with upper extremity hypertension, systolic murmur, and weak or absent femoral pulses. Ventricular septal defects are characterized by a loud, harsh, pansystolic murmur heard best at the lower left sternal border. Aortic stenosis has a systolic murmur.

10. **(1)** Mitral valve stenosis is a diastolic murmur of low intensity heard at the apex of the heart. Option #2 describes characteristics of a murmur with aortic stenosis. Option #3, a holosystolic murmur, is characteristic of mitral regurgitation,

which allows for backflow of blood from ventricles into the atrium. Option #4 best describes aortic regurgitation.

# Disorders

11. **(1)** A diagnosis of HTN from a single measurement of BP elevation should not be done. A minimum of three readings with an average systolic BP of 140 mm Hg and a diastolic BP of 90 mm Hg establishes the diagnosis. An average of two or more readings taken at each of two or more visits should follow an initial screening. The client should be seated with the arm at heart level. No caffeine or nicotine ingestion should be allowed 30 minutes prior to the reading. The room should be quiet a minimum of 5 minutes, and an appropriate cuff should be used. Another high reading should be confirmed within 2 months.

12. **(4)** The majority of cases of CHF in children result from congenital heart disease, and most occur during the first year of life. Although the clinical presentation of a child with congenital heart disease will vary with the specific defect, the clinical manifestations usually relate to the degree of CHF or cyanosis.

13. **(3)** Sinus or atrial tachycardia is characterized by a heart rate at or above 100, P waves are present for each QRS complex, the P-R interval is below 0.20, the T wave occurs after each QRS complex, and the beat is regular.

14. **(2)** Respiratory symptoms are predominant with clients in left-sided failure. Venous congestion and peripheral edema are associated with right-sided failure.

15. **(2)** Palpable carotid pulse with each compression is the best sign of effective CPR. The other answers are appropriate but not the best indicator of effective resuscitation efforts.

16. **(2)** Excess secretion of aldosterone predisposes to potassium excretion. Total body sodium content will be above normal, but the excessive secretion of antidiuretic hormone causes greater retention of water, diluting the serum level.

17. **(3)** The majority of cases of CHF in infants result from congenital heart disease during the first 12 months of life. Symptoms result from the decreased cardiac output and the infant's compensatory mechanisms. Symptoms include tachypnea, dyspnea, tachycardia, paleness, and easily fatigued. Additional symptoms include periorbital edema, hepatomegaly, difficulty feeding, and a persistent cough. Diaphoresis, central cyanosis, and peripheral edema are not necessarily associated with CHF, but may be manifestations of the underlying congenital heart defect of the infant.

18. **(4)** Common causes of chest pain include cardiac, chest wall, gastrointestinal, neurologic, and psychiatric causes. Ischemic heart disease, CHF, gastroesophageal reflux (GERD), and mitral valve prolapse (MVP) are more common in adults than children. Musculoskeletal problems such as costochondritis and idiopathic causes are more common in children. Idiopathic causes make up a large percentage of chest pain in children; symptoms appear to be self-limited and tend to diminish or resolve in 1 year. Cardiovascular causes in children are less common, but more serious if present and due to congenital heart lesions.

19. **(1)** Congenital heart disease is commonly classified as acyanotic or cyanotic. Cyanotic heart defects (right-to-left shunts) include tetralogy of Fallot, severe pulmonary stenosis, pulmonary atresia, tricuspid atresia, and transposition of the great vessels. Children with cyanotic heart disease develop polycythemia to increase the oxygen-carrying capacity of the blood. Additionally, the young child with a cyanotic heart defect should have a hemoglobin of at least 16 gm/dl.

20. **(1)** Although all of these conditions can lead to hypertension, the most common in infants and young children is secondary hypertension due to renal disease (i.e., glomerulonephritis, polycystic kidneys, nephrosis). Endocrine-induced hypertension is the second most common cause.

21. **(1)** The top two conditions known to play a causative role in the development of cardiovascular disease in children are untreated streptococcal infections involving group A β-hemolytic streptococcus (leads to cardiac valve problems) and Kawasaki disease (leads to coronary artery aneurysm).

22. **(4)** Options #1, #2, and #3 are considered unstable and acute and should be immediately referred to a pediatric cardiologist. Children with a murmur need to be further evaluated, but it is not considered an emergency as long as they are asymptomatic, have normal activity and exercise, and are growing normally.

23. **(3)** Procedures for which endocarditis prophylaxis is recommended include dental procedures known to include gingival bleeding, such as cleaning; tonsillectomy and/or adenoidectomy; and surgical procedures that involve respiratory mucosa. Endocarditis prophylaxis is not recommended for insertion of tympanostomy tubes, cardiac catheterization, simple dental procedures, or endotracheal intubation.

24. **(4)** For the child with a pacemaker, an electric shock may irreparably damage the pacemaker and thus immediate surgical replacement would be necessary. There is no risk of electromagnetic interference between the permanent pacemaker and household items such as electrical appliances, radios, electronic equipment, cellular phones, or microwave ovens. Microwave ovens and pacemakers have filtering systems that prevent interference with the pacemaker's function. Metal detectors have an electromagnetic field that could alter the pacemaker's function temporarily. In addition, the alarm will be set off as a result of the metal in the pacemaker.

25. **(1)** According to the Jones criteria, a diagnosis of rheumatic fever is highly likely if, in addition to two major manifestations (carditis, polyarthritis, Sydenham's chorea, erythema marginatum, and subcutaneous nodules), or one major and two minor manifestations (arthralgia, fever, elevated ESR, C-reactive protein, and prolonged P-R interval), there is evidence of a preceding group A streptococcus infection.

26. **(1)** The development of heart failure in the first few weeks of life, along with dyspnea, weak peripheral pulses, hepatomegaly, and grayish blue skin color, are characteristic of hypoplastic left heart syndrome. This is due to atresia of the aortic or mitral orifices and hypoplasia of the ascending aorta.

27. **(2)** Conservative management is indicated for high-normal elevations of blood pressure. Pharmacologic therapy may be useful but is not necessarily the initial recommendation. The STEP approach starts with a thiazide diuretic or adrenergic inhibitor, such as atenolol (Tenormin).

# Pharmacology

28. **(1)** Aldactone is a potassium-sparing diuretic. Parents should be instructed on signs of hyperkalemia.

29. **(1)** Secondary prevention, or preventing the recurrent attacks of acute rheumatic fever, is controversial. Some authorities identify the early 20s and 5 years since the last ARF attack as the criteria to stop the use of prophylactic penicillin, unless the client is at increased risk of exposure to streptococcal infections, such as schoolteachers or health professionals. Other authorities recommend lifelong prophylactic drug therapy. Although erythromycin is an alternative medication for penicillin-sensitive individuals, the dose in Option #2 is for a client having a dental or surgical procedure. The secondary prophylaxis dose for erythromycin is 250 mg PO bid.

30. **(2)** Nausea, vomiting, and anorexia are common side effect symptoms for many medications. The first-degree AV block is what confirms the ingestion of digoxin in this situation. Tricyclic antidepressant medication toxicity is characterized by agitation and anticholingeric symptoms. Lasix symptoms include hypokalemia, weakness, and cardiac arrhythmias. Aspirin toxicity symptoms include tinnitus, mental confusion, gastrointestinal symptoms, and rapid, deep respirations.

# 5

# Respiratory

## Physical Examination & Diagnostic Tests

1. The nurse practitioner knows that normal breath sounds that have a low pitch and soft intensity and are heard better on inspiration are called:

    1. Bronchial.

    2. Vesicular.

    3. Bronchovesicular.

    4. Rhonchi.

2. When auscultating for vocal resonance in a child with possible consolidation of lung tissue, the nurse practitioner hears "a-a-a" when the client says, "e-e-e." This is called:

    1. Tactile fremitus.

    2. Bronchophony.

    3. Whispered pectoriloquy.

    4. Egophony.

3. The nurse practitioner understands the following about hyperresonance in percussion of the lungs:

    1. It is a normal finding in the adult client.

    2. It occurs commonly in pediatric clients.

    3. It is characterized by soft intensity, high pitch, short duration, and extreme dull quality.

    4. It is characterized by loud intensity, high pitch, medium duration, and dull quality.

4. What is the correct procedure when percussing the chest?

    1. Start at the right upper side of the anterior chest and move to the left side.

    2. Begin at the upper left side of the posterior chest and compare to the respective anterior side, moving from front to back.

    3. Percuss systematically and symmetrically the anterior chest, moving from left to right side, then do the posterior chest.

    4. Percuss the posterior chest and then measure for diaphragmatic excursion on the anterior chest.

5. The nurse practitioner understands that pleural friction rubs are:

 1. Auscultated in the lower anterolateral chest.

 2. Heard best at the end of expiration.

 3. Characterized by a continuous, low-pitched snoring sound heard early in inspiration.

 4. Noted when the client says "e-e-e" and the examiner hears through the stethoscope "a-a-a."

6. When assessing for tactile fremitus, the nurse practitioner would place her hands over what area of the adolescent's chest?

 1. On the anterior chest at the level of the sixth intercostal space.

 2. At the level of bifurcation of the bronchi on the posterior chest wall.

 3. At the apex on the anterior chest wall.

 4. At the level of the diaphragm on the posterior chest wall.

7. An important anatomic landmark on the anterior thoracic wall is the angle of Louis. Where on the thorax is this landmark present?

 1. The mid-nipple line on either side of the manubrium.

 2. Bilaterally at the manubriosternal junction.

 3. Midline at the base of the suprasternal notch.

 4. Just below the clavicle but above the manubrium.

8. Cystic fibrosis is the preliminary diagnosis for a young girl who was brought to the clinic for evaluation. The test that will be used to rule out cystic fibrosis is:

 1. Hemoccult test.

 2. Sweat chloride test.

 3. Sputum culture and sensitivity.

 4. Glucose tolerance test.

9. When interpreting purified protein derivative (PPD) skin tests in children at a long-term juvenile detention facility, the nurse practitioner identifies positive results in individuals with:

 1. Redness or erythema at the site.

 2. A induration reaction of $\geq 5$ mm.

 3. A induration reaction of $\geq 10$ mm.

 4. A induration reaction extending to 15 mm.

## Disorders

10. A child has received a blunt trauma injury to his chest. An assessment finding that would be most indicative of further respiratory complications would be:

 1. Complaints of increased pain over the affected area.

 2. Oximetry readings consistently around 90%.

 3. Decreased breath sounds on the affected side.

 4. Fever of 102°F and increased sputum production.

11. A child is recovering from tuberculosis. What information should be included in a teaching plan for her home care?

 1. It is critical for the child to take medications at the prescribed time; do not skip doses or allow the supply to run out.

 2. Respiratory isolation procedures need to be carried out at home; the child should avoid contact with friends.

 3. It will be necessary for the parent to return the child to the clinic every week to have the child's sputum checked for viable bacteria.

 4. The child may experience a rash along with nausea and vomiting from the medications, and the parent should decrease the dosage if this occurs.

12. What would be a priority intervention for a school-aged child experiencing a respiratory arrest?

1. Start chest compressions at 15 compressions and 2 breaths.

2. Open the airway with a head tilt and chin lift.

3. Give oxygen via a rebreathing mask at 10 L/min.

4. Pinch the nose and give two breaths.

13. A child is severely dyspneic and the history strongly suggests the possibility of a foreign body in the bronchi. What observation would contribute to the documentation of this problem?

1. Unilateral retraction of the right chest wall.

2. Presence of crepitation on the anterior chest wall.

3. Retraction of the lower chest wall.

4. A friction rub heard over the area of the bronchi.

14. The nurse practitioner is assessing an adolescent who is complaining of shortness of breath and chest discomfort. His respirations are shallow and at a rate of 26. When evaluating the diaphragmatic excursion, it is determined that the diaphragm on the right is slightly higher than on the left side. The best interpretation of these findings is:

1. This is normal due to the liver on the right side.

2. There may be atelectasis in the right lower lobe.

3. Consolidation is present in the right lower lobe.

4. This indicates the presence of early stages of reactive airway disease.

15. A 15-year-old male comes to the office complaining of chest pain and shortness of breath. He states the problems started suddenly after running sprints in basketball practice. He states he has no past history of pulmonary problems. He is about 6 feet tall and weighs approximately 145 lb, his pulse rate is 118, his respiratory rate is 30, and there are decreased breath sounds and hyperresonance over the left lung. The best diagnosis for this client is:

1. Spontaneous pneumothorax.

2. Exercise-induced asthma.

3. Pulmonary edema.

4. Acute bronchiectasis.

16. A 16-year-old presents at the clinic with complaints of tingling in her face and hands, sudden shortness of breath, and vague chest discomfort. She appears very anxious and denies any history of respiratory problems. On examination, her hands are cool to touch; her vital signs are respirations 34, pulse regular at a rate of 100, blood pressure 104/68, and normal temperature. Respiratory examination reveals bilateral breath sounds with tachypnea, no adventitious sounds, and normal percussion and visual examination of the chest. The best immediate treatment is:

1. Rebreathing into a paper bag and encouraging controlled diaphragmatic breathing.

2. Albuterol (Proventil), two puffs with a metered-dose inhaler.

3. Oxygen at 4 L and arterial blood gases after 30 minutes.

4. Establish an IV, infuse 500 ml normal saline for volume depletion.

17. An 18-month-old infant is brought into the emergency room. He is awake, lethargic, and in severe respiratory distress. His mother states that he has not been sick and was playing on the floor when he suddenly began coughing, choking, and gagging. He has expiratory wheezes and there are decreased breath sounds over the right lower lobes. His respirations are 36, pulse is 130, and temperature is normal. A portable chest x-ray shows hyperinflation on expiratory views. The best treatment for this infant is:

1. Bronchoscopy as soon as possible.

2. Cool mist therapy with racemic epinephrine.

3. Antibiotics with chest physiotherapy.

4. Immediate endotracheal intubation and ventilation.

18. A 4-month-old client presents to the office with a history of several days of rhinorrhea, cough, a low-grade fever, and increased respiratory rate. The most likely diagnosis is:

    1. Croup.

    2. Epiglottitis.

    3. Tracheitis.

    4. Bronchiolitis.

19. An older adolescent comes to the clinic complaining of difficulty breathing, lethargy, and coughing up blood in his sputum. He has no history of chronic illness or major health problems. The nurse practitioner orders diagnostic tests to determine the problem. What diagnostic test results would require immediate treatment of this client?

    1. Positive sputum smear for acid-fast bacillus.

    2. Sputum culture positive for *Pneumocystis carinii*. normal/common resp tract organism

    3. Presence of hemolysis on complement fixation test.

    4. Oxygen saturation 94%, leukocyte count >5000 white blood cells (WBC)/mm$^3$.

20. During a physical exam of a 2-year-old diagnosed with possible cystic fibrosis, the child passes a stool. The nurse practitioner would expect the stool's appearance to be:

    1. Yellow and loose.

    2. Small and constipated.

    3. Green and odorous.

    4. Large and bulky.

21. The nurse practitioner understands the following about acute pneumonia:

    1. Viral pneumonia occurs primarily after age 5.

    2. Bacterial pneumonia is most common during the neonatal period.

    3. The most common cause of neonatal pneumonia is *Streptococcus pneumoniae*.

    4. Respiratory syncytial virus (RSV) is the major cause of pneumonia between 2 and 5 months of age.

22. The nurse practitioner knows that pneumonia can be distinguished from more common upper respiratory tract infections by the presence of:

    1. Tachypnea, crackles, hypoxemia, and cyanosis.

    2. Fever, rhinorrhea, fussiness, and cough.

    3. Coarse rhonchi, cough, tachycardia, and prostration.

    4. Wheezing, use of accessory muscles, fever, and cough.

23. The nurse practitioner understands the following about pertussis:

    1. Occurs by respiratory droplet infection.

    2. Has two phases, the catarrhal and paroxysmal. and convalescent

    3. Is associated with high temperatures and diminished breath sounds.

    4. Is treated with antiviral medications and humidification.

24. A 3-year-old client with a history of asthma presents to the office for evaluation by the nurse practitioner. The child has never used a peak flow meter. What quick tool can the nurse practitioner use to assess the severity of this child's distress?

    1. An arterial blood gas.

    2. The child's inability to complete a sentence.

    3. A chest x-ray.

    4. The presence of a runny nose.

25. Clinical signs and symptoms of late-phase asthma include:

    1. Bronchoconstriction refractory to bronchodilator therapy.

    2. Sneezing, watery eyes, and cough.

    3. Wheezing, increased sputum production.

    4. Bronchodilation secondary to release of histamine.

26. The nurse practitioner is assessing a child for asthma. What is a common clinical manifestation of asthma?

    1. Pruritis.

2. Diffuse crackles.

3. Nocturnal exacerbation.

4. Chronic hypoxemia.

27. A mother tells the nurse practitioner that her child has nocturnal asthma attacks. The nurse practitioner would expect the mother to explain that the attacks are the worst:

    1. At midnight.

    2. 2 hours after going to bed.

    3. Immediately after falling asleep.

    4. At 4 AM.

28. The nurse practitioner understands the following concerning tuberculosis:

    1. Infants are more likely than children to present with wheezing and rales.

    2. Older children develop disseminated disease and meningitis more often than infants.

    3. Affected infants and young children are more likely to have a PPD skin test induration of 15 mm or more.

    4. Adults are rarely the source of the disease when a child develops tuberculosis.

29. During a 4-month visit to the clinic for routine care, the mother reports that her infant, who was diagnosed with bronchopulmonary dysplasia (BPD), has been vomiting after each gastrostomy feeding. The nurse practitioner notes that the infant's weight gain is adequate and would recommend:

    1. Referral to the pediatrician for follow-up.

    2. Reduce the amount of formula for the gastrostomy feeding.

    3. Add 3 oz of Pedialyte for the next two feedings.

    4. Position the infant in a prone position after feedings with the head and trunk elevated.

30. A 3-year-old, who is up to date on his immunizations, is brought to the office by his mother with a fairly rapid onset of stridor and a high-pitched wheeze. In view of this information, the differential diagnosis that could be considered less likely than the others is:

1. Croup.

2. Foreign body aspiration.

3. Epiglottitis.

4. Bacterial tracheitis.

31. What is the etiologic agent in a child with acute epiglottis?

    1. Respiratory syncytial virus.

    2. *Haemophilus influenzae.*

    3. Parainfluenza virus.

    4. *Pneumococus.*

32. A restless, agitated, 1-year-old presents with a 2-day history of a brassy, harsh cough with difficulty breathing that worsens at night. Physical exam reveals diminished breath sounds bilaterally, harsh rhonchi, and crackles. The child's temperature is 101°F, pulse 178, and respirations 36. The nurse practitioner's diagnosis is:

    1. Acute epiglottis.

    2. Laryngotracheobronchitis.

    3. Pneumococcal pneumonia.

    4. Bronchiolitis.

# Pharmacology

33. The nurse practitioner is following up on a child who is experiencing acute asthmatic problems. Albuterol (Proventil) by metered-dose inhaler has been ordered as treatment. Which response would indicate to the nurse practitioner that the child understands how to take his medication?

    1. "I will take one puff of the medication and then wait a minute before taking the second puff."

    2. "I will take two puffs of the medication every 4 hours, even if I am not short of breath."

    3. "It is important for me to take this medication on a regular cycle to prevent future attacks."

    4. "I will take two puffs, one right after the other, whenever I begin to get short of breath."

34. An adolescent who was recently diagnosed with tuberculosis calls the clinic because her urine is reddish orange. She is taking isoniazid (Laniazid), rifampin (Rifadin), and pyrazinamide. An appropriate response for the nurse practitioner to make would be:

    1. "These are urinary tract infection symptoms; drink plenty of fluids."

    2. "This is a normal response to the rifampin."

    3. "Often this is an indication of liver toxicity. Stop the medications."

    4. "This is probably bleeding and you should see a physician immediately."

35. A 15-year-old female comes into the emergency room with complaints of extreme shortness of breath. She is confused and her past medical history is not available. Her vital signs are pulse 124, respirations 32, blood pressure 124/80, and temperature normal. Physical examination reveals diffuse expiratory wheezes, hyperresonance on percussion, and a prolonged expiratory phase. The best treatment for this client includes:

    1. Aminophylline by mouth.

    2. Beclomethasone (Beclovent) inhaler.

    3. Epinephrine by injection.

    4. Albuterol (Proventil) by nebulization therapy.

36. The recommended range for maintaining serum theophylline levels is:

    1. 0.05−2 μg/ml.

    2. 5−15 μg/ml.

    3. 20−25 μg/ml.

    4. 30−40 μg/ml.

37. An adolescent in a long-term juvenile detention facility whose roommate has been diagnosed as having active tuberculosis should be started on chemoprophylaxis:

    1. As soon as possible and initiated at the time of screening skin testing.

    2. In 72 hours after PPD skin test results are obtained.

    3. Only if PPD skin test results are positive.

    4. In 3 months if the repeated skin test is positive.

38. Which medication is most effective in promoting a decrease in airway inflammation as well as providing long-term medication coverage in a child with asthma?

    1. Isoetharine (Bronkometer).

    2. Beclomethasone dipropionate (Vanceril, Beclovent).

    3. Albuterol (Proventil, Ventolin).

    4. Pirbuterol (Maxair).

39. The nurse practitioner is planning prophylactic treatment for a client with asthma. What is the best medication to use for the asthmatic client who is not currently experiencing an exacerbation?

    1. Antibiotics.

    2. Inhaled glucocorticoids.

    3. β-Agonist.

    4. Methylacholine challenge.

40. Children with asthma need to be instructed to:

    1. Begin their inhaled steroids as soon as symptoms appear.

    2. Using the metered dose inhaler, take two puffs of the $\beta_2$-agonist prn.

    3. Use their inhaled steroids when they experience bronchospasm.

    4. Start their antibiotic regimen when they experience bronchospasm.

41. The nurse practitioner understands that an appropriate medication regimen for a child with tuberculosis is:

    1. Single-drug therapy with rifampin (Rifadin).

    2. Combination therapy with streptomycin, pyrazinamide, and rimantadine (Flumadine).

3. Combination therapy with isoniazide, pyrazinamide, and rifampin.

4. Single-drug therapy with pyrimethamine (Fansidar).

42. During a routine well-child exam of a 4-year-old, the nurse practitioner learns that the paternal grandmother has just been diagnosed with active tuberculosis. The mother states that the grandmother had stayed in their home for a week during the summer. The child has no signs of tuberculosis and has a negative PPD. The nurse practitioner should:

1. Prescribe no medications, but schedule a repeat PPD in 2 months.

2. Administer 1 ml gamma globulin IM.

3. Start the child on a combination of isoniazid and rifampin therapy for 15 months.

4. Start the child on isoniazid therapy for 3 months and then re-evaluate.

43. An adolescent presents in the clinic with a dry, hacking, nonproductive cough that is interfering with her sleep. The nurse practitioner would encourage the client to purchase an over-the-counter preparation that contains:

1. Pseudoephedrine.

2. Phenylpropanolamine.

3. Guaifenesin.

4. Dextromethorphan.

44. Indications for antibiotic use in a child with asthmatic bronchitis would include:

1. History of two episodes in 4 months.

2. Rhinitis and a productive cough.

3. High fever and rales.

4. Low-grade fever and sibilant wheezes.

45. A 10-year-old on isoniazid (INH) prophylactically for exposure to tuberculosis complains of tingling and numbness in his feet, a rash, and diarrhea. Management would be based on:

1. Avoidance of tyramine- and histamine-containing foods.

2. Addition of pyridoxine to the diet.

3. Changing the INH to rifampin (Rifadin).

4. Evaluation for hepatic impairment.

46. What is the initial treatment of choice for children diagnosed with bronchiolitis?

1. Increase fluids; albuterol (Ventolin) in saline inhalation every 4–6 hours.

2. Prednisolone (Pediapred) immediately and continue over 3–5 days.

3. Diphenhydramine HCl (Benadryl) every 4–6 hours as long as symptoms persist.

4. Amoxicillin over 10–14 days and aerosol humidification.

47. A 10-year-old boy is experiencing problems with wheezing, coughing, and shortness of breath about 4 hours after basketball practice. He has normal respirations and only experiences the problems after exercise. He is experiencing no other respiratory problems and the physical exam is within normal limits. What is the treatment of choice for this child?

1. Albuterol (Ventolin) 20–30 minutes prior to exercise.

2. Cromolyn sodium (Intal) two puffs each morning.

3. Theophylline (Theo-Dur) PO bid.

4. Beclomethasone (Beclovent) two puffs 3–4 times daily.

48. Which medication would the nurse practitioner prescribe for an infant with RSV bronchiolitis?

1. Amoxicillin (Amoxil).

2. Ribavirin (Virazole).

3. Ceftriaxone (Rocephin).

4. Vancenase (Vanceril).

49. Which statement is correct concerning montelukast (Singulair)?

    1. Recommended for the treatment of asthma in infants and toddlers.

    2. Effective in the primary treatment of an acute asthma attack.

    3. Useful as monotherapy for exercise-induced asthma in the adolescent; has minimal side effects.

    4. Acts as a leukotriene receptor antagonist in the treatment of asthma in children ages 6–14 years.

50. Which statement is correct concerning the nonsedating antihistamine astemizole (Hismanal)?

    1. Indicated for children under the age of 12.

    2. May cause ventricular arrhythmias (torsade de pointes).

    3. May be taken concomitantly with erythromycin.

    4. Rarely causes syncope or heart block.

# 5 ⟩ Answers & Rationales

## Physical Examination & Diagnostic Tests

1. **(2)** The sounds heard over normal lung tissue are called vesicular breath sounds. The inspiratory phase of the vesicular breath sound is heard better than the expiratory phase and is about 2.5 times longer for these low-pitched, soft sounds. Bronchial breath sounds are normally heard over the trachea and usually indicate pathology. Bronchial breath sounds are high-pitched, loud sounds with a shortened inspiratory and lengthened expiratory phase. Bronchovesicular breath sounds have an intermediate pitch and intensity with equal duration of expiratory and inspiratory sounds heard mainly over the second interspace anteriorly and between the scapulae posteriorly. Rhonchi are abnormal breath sounds that are low pitched with a snoring quality.

2. **(4)** Tactile fremitus is a palpable vibration of the thoracic wall that is produced when the client speaks. Bronchophony is the increase in loudness and clarity of vocal resonance. Whispered pectoriloquy is exaggerated bronchophony and is heard through a stethoscope when the client whispers a series of words (e.g., "ninety-nine"). In egophony the spoken voice has a nasal or bleating quality when heard through a stethoscope and the spoken "e-e-e" sounds like "a-a-a."

3. **(2)** Hyperresonance is an abnormal percussion tone in adults but occurs normally in a child's lung. It is characterized by very loud intensity, very low pitch, long duration, and a booming quality.

4. **(3)** Both the anterior and posterior chest are to be percussed systematically and symmetrically, moving from left to right. Diaphragmatic excursion is usually only measured on the posterior chest.

5. **(1)** Most often heard in the lower anterolateral thorax, pleural friction rubs are loud, dry, creaking or grating sounds produced by the rubbing together of inflamed and roughened pleural surfaces, and are heard best during the latter part of inspiration and the beginning of expiration. Option #3 is characteristic of sonorous rhonchi.

6. **(2)** The bifurcation of the trachea or bronchi on the posterior chest wall is the best area for assessment of tactile fremitus. Care should be taken to avoid the area over the scapula.

7. **(2)** This landmark can be used to determine the position of the second rib and intercostal space and corresponding spaces below that level. It is a visible and palpable angle of the sternum at the point where the second rib attaches to the sternum.

8. **(2)** A sweat chloride test is positive for cystic fibrosis due to the abnormal amount of sodium chloride in the sweat. A hemoccult is a test for blood in the stool. Sputum culture and sensitivity are performed to determine what medication is effective against as organism. The glucose tolerance test is performed to diagnose diabetes.

9. **(3)** Positive interpretations of PPD skin test results are as follows:

| Induration | Positive in: |
| --- | --- |
| ≥ 5 mm | Individuals with human immunodeficiency virus (HIV) infection |
| | Recent close contact with individuals with active tuberculosis (TB) |
| | Individuals with chest x-ray indicating healed TB |
| ≥ 10 mm | Medically underserved |
| | IV drug users |
| | Clients in long-term care facilities |
| ≥ 15 mm | All individuals |

# Disorders

10. **(3)** The most common respiratory complication after a traumatic injury to the chest is pneumothorax caused from a fractured rib. Oximetry readings at 90% and increased pain are expected at this point and may not be indicative of a problem.

11. **(1)** On discharge, a client must understand the importance of taking medications as prescribed. If doses are missed, it will increase the mutation of the tubercle bacillus and decrease the effectiveness of the medication. Respiratory isolation at home is not necessary and, if she experiences problems of rash, nausea, and vomiting, the parents should contact her health care provider. Weekly sputum checks are not necessary.

12. **(2)** According to the American Heart Association, the protocol for CPR (rescue breathing) due to respiratory arrest would be to open the airway by tilting the head and lifting the chin.

13. **(1)** The most common area for a foreign body obstruction is the right bronchi; this will produce a unilateral retraction of the right chest wall. Retraction of the lower chest occurs with lower respiratory problems such as asthma. A pleural friction rub is heard when there is inflammation between the visceral and parietal pleura. Crepitation is present when air is leaking into the subcutaneous tissue.

14. **(1)** This is a normal finding due to the bulk of the liver. Atelectasis and consolidation will present with normal diaphragmatic movement but with dullness to percussion over the affected area. Obstructive lung disease will result in hyperresonance and limited diaphragmatic excursion but it will be bilateral.

15. **(1)** Spontaneous pneumothorax occurs in healthy, thin young adults, especially after strenuous exercise; predominant symptoms include sudden pain and dyspnea. The clinical hallmark of asthma is wheezing; with pulmonary edema there is frequently coughing, frothy sputum, and crackles heard on auscultation. Bronchiectasis is most often chronic and is characterized by moist crackles and wheezing on auscultation; cough is usually present.

16. **(1)** The situation described is hyperventilation. By slowing the breathing and breathing into a paper bag, the carbon dioxide levels will be restored and the acid–base problem resolved. Albuterol, oxygen, arterial blood gases (ABGs), and IV fluids are not appropriate initial treatment.

17. **(1)** The child had the symptoms and history that are consistent with a partial airway obstruction from aspiration of a foreign body. Direct laryngoscopy or bronchoscopy are necessary to remove the foreign body. Chest physiotherapy may dislodge the object and force it further into the airway. Antibiotics and epinephrine are not going to be effective. There is no need to intubate the infant if the foreign body can be removed.

18. **(4)** Croup, epiglottitis, and tracheitis are all middle respiratory tract infections with a rapid onset. Bronchiolitis is a lower respiratory tract infection that has a more gradual onset and no "barking" sound to the cough.

19. **(1)** The positive sputum for acid-fast bacillus is indicative of active tuberculosis. The *P. carinii* is a common organism in healthy respiratory tracts; it becomes a problem if the client is immunocompromised. Hemolysis on a complement fixation test is a negative finding. The oxygen saturation is low, but the leukocyte count is within normal ranges; therefore treatment of this condition is not as important as for the tuberculosis.

20. **(4)** In cystic fibrosis the stools are large, bulky, and foul smelling (steatorrhea). Yellow stools are indicative of liver or gallbladder problems. Green stools often indicate a rapid transit time and may be associated with infection.

21. **(4)** Viruses are the most common cause of pneumonia between 2 and 5 years of age. RSV is the major cause of pneumonia between 2 and 5 months of age. *Streptococcus pneumoniae* is the most common bacterial agent, and most bacterial pneumonias become less common after the neonatal period.

22. **(1)** Acute respiratory infections are the most common illnesses in the pediatric client, with acute pneumonia accounting for only a small percentage (10%–15%). However, pneumonia has significant morbidity and mortality among children. It is distinguished by the presence of lower respiratory tract signs (e.g., tachypnea, crackles, hypoxemia, and cyanosis) plus a pulmonary infiltrate on chest x-ray.

23. **(1)** Pertussis is characterized by a persistent "whooping" type cough, afebrile, and classically presents in three stages— catarrhal, paroxysmal, and convalescent. It is highly communicable by respiratory droplet infection especially during the catarrhal stage. Incubation period is 7–10 days after exposure. It is treated preferably with a macrolide (erythromycin, azithromycin, etc.) for 14 days or TMP-SMX, as an alternative medication.

24. **(2)** In children too young to properly use a peak flow meter, the inability to cry or complete a sentence may indicate an acute asthma attack. An arterial blood gas study is usually not performed in office settings, and a chest x-ray will most likely agitate the child and take too long to process.

25. **(1)** Late-phase asthma occurs at 6–12 hours after the initial or acute bronchoconstrictive phase. The inflammatory response is the result of mast cell degranulation and release of histamine. Histamine acts on the lung by causing bronchoconstriction, vascular permeabilty, and vasodilatation. In late-phase asthma, bronchoconstriction is refractory to most bronchodilator therapy.

26. **(3)** Nocturnal exacerbation of asthma is a common clinical sign. It is linked to the variation in circulating catecholamines and vagal tone. Chronic hypoxemia and diffuse crackles are seen in the child with chronic bronchitis. Pruritus is often seen in contact allergic reactions.

27. **(4)** Nocturnal asthma attacks are generally the worst at 4 AM when bronchial constriction occurs due to changes in the circadian rhythm that affect bronchial reactivity.

28. **(1)** In addition to more symptoms of wheezing and rales, infants are more likely to develop disseminated disease such as meningitis and to have a negative PPD skin test. Usually, the transmission of the disease can be traced to an affected adult living in the household.

29. **(4)** Maintaining a high caloric intake is important in the care of infants with BPD to promote growth and nourishment of developing lung tissue. Sometimes, infants have gastroesophageal reflux (GER) after feedings. Initially positioning should be tried; then feedings may be thickened or given in smaller amounts more frequently. If the problem persists or if the weight gain is not adequate, then referral to a pediatrician is indicated.

30. **(3)** If this child is up to date on his immunizations, he should have had his *Haemophilus influenzae* type b vaccine (HIB), the most common cause of epiglottitis. A dramatic decline in the incidence of epiglottitis and *H. influenzae* type b infections is associated closely with the history of the HIB vaccines. Considering the age of this child and the suddenness of the onset, the most likely diagnosis is foreign body aspiration.

31. **(2)** The etiologic agent is *Haemophilus influenzae*. Respiratory syncytial virus (RSV) is the etiologic agent for bronchiolitis. *Pneumococcus* is present in pneumococcal pneumonia cases. Parainfluenza virus is found in most cases of croup (i.e., laryngotracheobronchitis [LTB]).

32. **(2)** These are classic symptoms of LTB. There is no drooling, high fever, aphonia, and severe respiratory distress, which are associated with acute epiglottis. The expiratory phase is prolonged and there is no wheezing in bronchiolitis due to RSV. With pneumonia, there would be purulent sputum, chills, and use of the accessory muscles of breathing.

# Pharmacology

33. **(1)** In order for the medication to be most effective, there needs to be a 1-minute time lapse between the two puffs of medication. The first puff will open the upper airways. This will allow more effective penetration of the lower tract with the second puff of medication.

34. **(2)** The client should not stop taking the medications as this is a common side effect of rifampin. Also, soft contact lenses may become discolored.

35. **(4)** A β-agonist (albuterol) is the first line of treatment to decrease airflow obstruction. Aminophylline by mouth would take too long to be effective. Epinephrine is used predominantly for anaphylactic reactions. Beclovent is a steroid inhaler that is most effective when used prophylcatically rather than in acute episodes.

36. **(2)** Therapeutic plasma levels range from 5 to 15 μg/ml. Drug levels of ≥20 μg/ml are associated with toxicity.

37. **(1)** Chemoprophylaxis is initiated at the time of the screening skin testing. Skin testing should be repeated in 3 months if initial test results are negative. If the second skin testing is negative, chemoprophylaxis can be stopped.

38. **(2)** Beclomethasone dipropionate is a long-acting corticosteroid that stabilizes mast cells and greatly reduces mast cell degranulation when exposed to allergens. All of the other medications are bronchodilators used for rapid reversal of bronchospasm.

39. **(2)** Treatment of the client with asthma includes inhaled glucocorticoids for their anti-inflammatory effects. Antibiotics are indicated if there is a concurrent infection such as acute bronchitis. $\beta_2$-Agonists are used for their bronchodilator effects and rapid onset of action. Methylacholine challenge is used in the diagnosis of asthma.

40. **(2)** Children with asthma should be instructed to keep their inhaled $\beta_2$-agonists with them at all times in case of bronchospasm and use them prn. The $\beta_2$-agonists are effective in reversing bronchospasm. Inhaled steroids are long acting and will not give immediate relief; therefore, clients should be instructed to use them regularly as prescribed and use their inhaled $\beta_2$-agonist prn. Beginning antibiotics is not indicated for acute bronchospasm.

41. **(3)** These are the common drugs used for combination therapy for the treatment of tuberculosis in children. Rimantadine is an antiviral; Fansidar is an antimalarial. Single-drug therapy is not indicated due to the virulence of the tubercle bacillus.

42. **(4)** Close contact of clients with an active case of tuberculosis should be placed on isoniazid single-drug therapy, even if the tuberculin skin test is negative. This early treatment will destroy the tubercle bacillus before hypersensitivity develops. The isoniazid should be continued for 3 months for those people whose skin test remains negative and there is no evidence of disease. If there is a positive skin test conversion, isoniazid (10–20 mg/kg) should be continued for 1 year. If the child develops symptoms of tuberculosis, he should be given isoniazid and rifampin (10 mg/kg) for 1 year.

43. **(4)** Dextromethorphan is specific for control of coughing. Guaifenesin is an expectorant, and Options #1 and #2 are decongestants to decrease nasal and upper respiratory congestion.

44. **(3)** Rhinitis and a productive cough are common and not cause for concern unless the mucus begins to change color and is accompanied by a high fever. The wheezes are also common, if the mucus is loose. A high fever and rales indicate further deterioration and possible bacterial infection.

45. **(2)** Pyridoxine (vitamin $B_6$) is added to prevent peripheral neuropathy. Tyramine- and histamine-containing foods such as tuna, aged cheese, and yeast vitamin supplements cause interaction with the monoamine oxidase (MAO) inhibitors. Anorexia, jaundice, malaise, and fatigue would be signs of hepatic involvement.

46. **(1)** Bronchodilators are frequently effective for acute episodes. Antibiotics and antihistamines are not effective and should not be used. The condition is usually treated symptomatically. If the child does not improve, consult a physician.

47. **(1)** Medications should be taken only when the child is going to exercise and anticipates respiratory difficulty. Intal and Beclovent are steroids and do not provide immediate relief, and theophylline should be avoided unless symptoms get progressively worse

and cannot be controlled with inhalation therapy.

48. **(2)** Antiviral medications such as ribavirin (Virazole) are indicated in the early course of treatment with a child with RSV bronchiolitis who is under 2 years of age. Antibiotics are not indicated unless there is a secondary bacterial infection. Aerosolized bronchodilators are frequently used; oral steroids usually are not.

49. **(4)** Antiasthmatic medication that acts as a leukotriene receptor antagonist in the treatment of asthma is recommended for children ages 6–14 years. It is not indicated in the primary treatment of an acute asthma attack. It is not recommended as monotherapy for exercise-induced asthma in the adolescent. Side effects include headache, fatigue, fever, gastrointestinal upset, laryngitis, and pharyngitis.

50. **(2)** Hismanal (along with the former Seldane) can cause ventricular arrhythmias (torsade de pointes). This medication is not recommended for children. Concomitant use with erythromycin or ketoconazole may affect its metabolism. If syncope occurs, the drug is to be immediately discontinued.

# 6

# Immune & Allergy

## Physical Examination & Diagnostic Tests

1. When taking the history of a child with known allergies, what is the most important information to determine?

   1. Reaction associated with each allergen.

   2. Drug allergies.

   3. Food allergies.

   4. Environmental exposure.

2. Which test is used to test determine the concentration of gamma globulins that contain most of the immunoglobulins?

   1. Immunofixation electrophoresis.

   2. Complement fixation. *C₃,C₄,C₅₀*

   3. Protein electrophoresis. *Ig E,G,M,A*

   4. Antinuclear antibody. *ANA*

3. Which tests are appropriate for the nurse practitioner to order in an initial work-up for asymptomatic clients at risk for human immunodeficiency virus (HIV)?

   1. CD4 count, HIV enzyme-linked immunosorbent assay (ELISA).

2. Serology for cytomegalovirus, herpes simplex virus, Epstein-Barr virus.

3. HIV ELISA and Western blot.

4. Hepatitis screen and Western blot.

4. The nurse practitioner would anticipate which laboratory finding in a client with joint pain, "butterfly rash," photosensitivity, weight loss, and fever?

   1. Presence of antinuclear antibodies.

   2. Negative serum complement level.

   3. Increased red blood cell (RBC) and white blood cell (WBC) count.

   4. Glycosuria.

5. When assessing a child for angioedema, the nurse practitioner would examine the:

   1. Neck and ears.

   2. Heart sounds.

   3. Abdomen.

   4. Eyes and mouth.

6. Adolescents who believe they have been exposed to HIV should have an HIV antibody test how soon after the exposure?

   1. The next day and 2 months later.

   2. 6 months after exposure and again at 12 months.

   3. 6–12 weeks after exposure and again at 6 months.

   4. 4 weeks and 12 weeks.

7. The most reliable test for the presence of specific immunoglobulin E (IgE) antibody is:

   1. Skin testing.

   2. Radioallergosorbent testing (RAST).

   3. Smears for eosinophils.

   4. Complete blood count (CBC).

8. To diagnose allergic rhinitis in the primary care office setting, the nurse practitioner would consider performing:

   1. A nasal smear for eosinophils.

   2. A total serum IgE.

   3. Skin testing.

   4. Radioallergosorbent tests (RAST).

9. The nurse practitioner is evaluating the tuberculin skin test on an immunocompetent child who has no risk factors for tuberculosis. The purified protein derivative test (PPD) is considered positive when it measures:

   1. 5 mm.

   2. 10 mm.

   3. 15 mm.

   4. 20 mm.

10. A new mother tells the clinic nurse that her infant was born HIV-positive. She asks the nurse how long her baby has to live. The nurse's response would be based on the knowledge that:

    1. The antibodies present in the baby's blood may reflect the antibodies received from the mother at the time of birth.

    2. If antibodies are present at birth, the baby has acquired immunodeficiency syndrome (AIDS) in an active form.

    3. Since the baby is HIV positive, the child will develop full-blown AIDS within 3 years.

    4. The antibodies detected at birth indicate presence of the HIV; the test does not indicate when the child will develop AIDS.

11. Diagnostic studies used in the differential diagnosis of systemic lupus erythematosus (SLE) include:

    1. CBC, $SMA_{12}$, and erythrocyte sedimentation rate (ESR).

    2. Chest radiograph and coagulation profile.

    3. Antinuclear antibody (ANA), ESR, and C-reactive protein.

    4. CBC, urinalysis, chest radiograph.

# Disorders

12. Parent education regarding common antigens of anaphylaxis includes:

    1. Extreme weather.

    2. Egg albumin.

    3. Pungent odors.

    4. Animal dandruff.

13. The nurse practitioner understands that an HIV infection results in a reduction of:

    1. Helper T cells.

    2. Suppressor T cells.

    3. Killer T cells.

    4. Suppressor B cells.

14. After a repeat HIV antibody test, an adolescent continues to test positive but is asymptomatic. The nurse practitioner understands which of the following about possible transmission of the virus by the client?

    1. The client is infectious when symptoms are active.

2. The client is infectious for life.

3. The dormant virus is not infectious while the client is asymptomatic and the T cell count is high.

4. Laboratory tests should be done monthly to identify the infectious periods of the disease process.

15. An adolescent has just received news of a positive HIV test. She does not want her sexual partner to be informed. What is the most appropriate response to her decision?

    1. Respect for her decision since she is the client.

    2. Letting her know that you have a legal responsibility to inform her partner.

    3. Counseling her about your ethical responsibility to inform all sexual partners.

    4. Noting her decision in the record for future reference.

16. An adolescent presenting with complaints of fatigue, malaise, arthralgias, oral ulcers, malar rash, and a positive ANA would most likely be diagnosed as having:

    1. Rheumatoid arthritis.

    2. Fibromyalgia.

    3. Scleroderma.

    4. Systemic lupus erythematosus.

17. A client presents with sneezing, watery eyes, postnasal drip, full head, and sore throat. The best diagnosis for this client is:

    1. Acute bronchitis.

    2. Allergic rhinitis.

    3. Asthma exacerbation.

    4. Influenza.

18. The erythematous confluent macular eruption of the face known as the butterfly rash is characteristic of:

    1. Allergic drug eruption.

    2. Systemic lupus erythematosus.

    3. Rosacea.

    4. Seborrheic dermatitis.

19. The release of histamine results in:

    1. Bronchospasm, vasodilation, and vascular permeability.

    2. Bronchodilatation, vasodilatation, and vascular permeability.

    3. Smooth muscle contraction, decreased vascular permeability, and vasoconstriction.

    4. Pain, increased vascular permeability, and bronchodilatation.

20. The nurse practitioner is discussing general health care with an adolescent who is in remission for SLE. Important points to include are:

    1. Avoid getting pregnant.

    2. Decrease physical and psychological stress.

    3. Avoid isometric and aerobic exercise.

    4. Maintain diet low in fat and carbohydrates.

21. When teaching a family about risk factors and prevention of transmission of HIV, which statement is most appropriate?

    1. HIV can be transmitted by casual kissing.

    2. Unprotected oral sex with an infected partner is not advised.

    3. Sharing a room with an HIV-positive person increases the risk of exposure to HIV.

    4. Using the same bathroom as an infected family member puts you at risk of exposure to HIV.

22. Signs and symptoms that alert the nurse practitioner to identify an adolescent who is at an increased risk for HIV infection include:

    1. Night sweats.

    2. Malaise and fatigue.

    3. Frequent sexually transmitted diseases.

    4. Swollen glands and diarrhea.

23. HIV is classified as a:

    1. Cytomegalovirus.

    2. Herpetic virus.

    3. Papillomavirus.

    4. Retrovirus.

24. The most frequently occurring symptoms of SLE are:

    1. Splenomegaly and Raynaud's syndrome.

    2. Pulmonary effusions and hepatomegaly.

    3. Butterfly rash on the face and lymphadenopathy.

    4. Fever, arthritis, arthralgia, and weight loss.

25. A systemic IgE-mediated antigen–antibody response resulting in a life-threatening massive release of mediators is:

    1. Generalized seizures.

    2. Allergic rhinitis.

    3. Anaphylaxis.

    4. Status asthmaticus.

26. Following a bone marrow transplant (BMT), the nurse practitioner can expect the peak onset of an acute graft-versus-host disease (GVHD) to occur:

    1. Between 10 and 15 days posttransplant.

    2. Between 30 and 50 days posttransplant.

    3. Between 1 and 5 days posttransplant.

    4. At 100 days posttransplant.

27. A child has a history of recent BMT. The nurse practitioner identifies sign and symptoms of GVHD to include:

    1. Fever, headache, and mental status changes.

    2. Chills, fever, and urticaria over flank area.

    3. Increased serum bilirubin, maculopapular rash, and green, watery diarrhea.

    4. Decreased RBC, hematocrit, and hemoglobin; petechiae, and increased bleeding tendencies.

28. The pathogenesis of SLE is characterized by autoantibody development. This results in:

    1. Increased T suppressor cell.

    2. B-cell decrease.

    3. Polyclonal hypogammaglobulinemia.

    4. Decreased T suppressor cells and inhibited cell activity.

29. The cell responsible for the activation of the immune response are the:

    1. Band neutrophils.

    2. T4 lymphocytes. (T helper)

    3. Segmented neutrophils.

    4. B lymphocytes.

30. A 19-year-old male presents with breathlessness, weight loss, nonproductive cough, temperature of 38°C (100.4°F), pulse 124, respirations 36, blood pressure 120/78, and a history of a positive HIV serum test. Based on this information, what is the most accurate diagnosis?

    1. *Klebsiella pneumonia.*

    2. Kaposi's sarcoma.

    3. *Pneumocystis carinii* pneumonia.

    4. Lymphoma.

31. A child is brought into the clinic and the family states he has a history of anaphylactic reactions. What signs and symptoms indicate to the nurse practitioner that the client is experiencing another reaction?

    1. Cough, wheezing, and hives.

    2. Severe malaise, pallor, stridor, and dyspnea.

    3. Anxiety, nasal congestion, and tachycardia.

    4. Rhinorrhea, nausea, and gastrointestinal (GI) cramping.

32. A nurse at the clinic experiences a needle stick from an adolescent with known hepatitis. What immunoglobulin (Ig) should be administered to provide passive immunity?

    1. IgE.

    2. IgA.

3. IgG.

4. IgC.

33. Which sign and/or symptom is indicative of a type I hypersensitivity reaction?

1. Contact dermatitis. *Type IV*

2. Immediate wheal-and-flare reaction. *Type I*

3. Hematuria. *Type II*

4. High fever. *Type III*

34. Which clients are at risk for developing HIV/AIDS?

1. Immunocompromised clients.

2. Sexually active teenagers.

3. Family of an HIV individual.

4. Marijuana users.

35. A 12-month-old infant was exposed to hepatitis A and received gammaglobulin therapy. What is important to tell the mother?

1. The child has been immunized against hepatitis A.

2. The child should not receive the scheduled dose of varicella at the 12 month vaccination.

3. Maintain body fluid precautions with the child.

4. Watch the child for easy bruising or signs of bleeding.

36. When assessing a client for SLE, what ophthalmologic findings would the nurse practitioner determine to be consistent with this condition?

1. Conjunctival hemorrhages.

2. Conjunctivitis.

3. Brushfield's spots.

4. Arteriovenous (AV) nicking.

37. What information does the nurse practitioner include in the education for the child with allergic rhinitis?

1. Monitor air quality and the allergy index.

2. Use a surgical-type mask when going outdoors.

3. Remain inside during allergy season.

4. Avoid playing outdoors near a garden.

38. Which statement is true regarding latex allergy?

1. It usually produces symptoms of contact dermatitis and allergic rhinorrhea.

2. It is a progressive disease that worsens with continued exposure.

3. It only affects less than 5% of the health care population.

4. It is an autoimmune response.

39. Children who have chronic allergic rhinitis often present with clinical symptoms that include:

1. Mouth breathing and nasal polyps.

2. Allergic shiners and Dennie lines.

3. Thick nasal discharge and sneezing.

4. Flushed face and fever.

40. Common sites for adolescent atopic dermatitis are:

1. Cheeks, forehead, and scalp.

2. Wrists, ankles, and antecubital fossae.

3. Antecubital fossae, face, neck, and back.

4. Palmar creases and extensor surface of legs.

# Pharmacology

41. Drugs that have been associated with a lupus-like syndrome include:

1. Sulfonamides (Septra DS), penicillin (Pen VK, Penicillin G).

2. Progestin/estrogen combination of oral contraceptives.

3. Nonsteroidal anti-inflammatory drugs (Motrin).

4. Procainamide (Pronestyl), hydralazine (Apresoline).

42. The clinic is notified that a child is being brought in with a bee sting and that the child is having difficulty breathing. Which medication should the nurse practitioner have available for the child's initial care?

    1. Lidocaine topical ointment.

    2. Epinephrine.

    3. Prednisone.

    4. Benadryl elixir.

43. The standard drug used for malaria prophylaxis is:

    1. Ampicillin (Polycillin, Omnipen).

    2. Doxycycline (Vibramycin).

    3. Ceftriaxone (Rocephin).

    4. Chloroquine phosphate (Aralen).

44. Treatment for allergic rhinitis includes:

    1. Antihistamines, corticosteroids, and environmental control.

    2. Antibiotics, antihistamines, analgesics, and allergen control.

    3. Cholinergic agents, antibiotics, and analgesics.

    4. Nasal saline, corticosteroids, and antibiotics.

45. A medication frequently used for the prophylaxis as well as initial treatment of *Pneumocystis carinii* pneumonia (PCP) is:

    1. Fluconazole (Diflucan).

    2. Amphotericin B (Fungizone).

    3. Trimethoprim-sulfamethoxazole (Septra, Bactrim).

    4. Acyclovir (Zovirax).

46. When instructing the adolescent with allergic rhinitis about the use of topical nasal decongestants, it is important for them to understand:

    1. The condition is self-limiting and will resolve in a matter of weeks whether or not the child is re-exposed to the allergen.

    2. Topical nasal decongestant used continuously for >3 days can result in a worsening of the symptoms.

    3. It is not necessary to avoid exposure to the allergen once therapy has been initiated.

    4. Allergic rhinitis is only seen in the spring and fall; the condition only requires treatment during these seasons.

47. The major advantage to use of second-generation antihistamines such as astemizole (Hismanal) and loratadine (Claritin) is:

    1. Decreased cost.

    2. Increased anticholinergic activity.

    3. Delayed absorption.

    4. Does not cross the blood–brain barrier.

48. What is the desired action of sympathomimetics (adrenergics) when used in the treatment of allergic rhinitis?

    1. Promote vasoconstriction in nasal mucosa.

    2. Block mast cell degranulation.

    3. Decrease the effect of histamines.

    4. Increase degranulation and end-organ response.

49. Cromolyn sodium is used to:

    1. Reduce the histamine load.

    2. Antagonize the effects of histamine.

    3. Stabilize the mast cell membrane.

    4. Reduce antiemetic activity.

50. A primary advantage of using loratadine (Claritin) in treating an adolescent with seasonal allergies is that it:

    1. Is supplied as an enteric-coated pill.

    2. May be prescribed as once-a-day dosing.

    3. Costs considerably less than other medications.

    4. Effectively decreases nasal secretions.

51. What medications are the choice of treatment in secondary therapy for the child with an anaphylactic reaction?

    1. Antibiotics and anticholinergics.

    2. Nonsteroidal anti-inflammatory drugs (NSAIDs).

    3. Decongestants and expectorants.

    4. Antihistamines and corticosteroids.

52. An appropriate antihistamine to recommend for a child with allergic rhinitis is:

    1. Diphenhydramine (Benadryl).

    2. Dextromethorphan (Benylin).

    3. Guaifenesin (Robitussin).

    4. Brompheniramine (Dimetane).

53. A child who weighs 30 lb (13.6 kg) arrives in the office with a complaint of an allergic reaction to peanuts. The child has hives on most of her body and is beginning to wheeze; she is in acute distress. The nurse practitioner administers:

    1. Diphenhydramine (Benadryl) 50 mg PO.

    2. Diphenhydramine (Benadryl) 25 mg PO.

    3. Epinephrine (adrenaline) 0.14 ml of a 1:1000 solution SQ.

    4. Epinephrine (adrenaline) 0.3 ml of a 1:1000 solution SQ.

# Answers & Rationales

## Physical Examination & Diagnostic Tests

1. **(1)** The reaction to each allergen is important to know. Often parents will indicate that their children have a reaction to a particular food or medication, such as nausea, stomach pain, or diarrhea, and consider it an allergy. The signs and symptoms of the reaction, speed of onset, how long it lasts, and what successful treatment has been used in the past is important information. Both drug and food allergies should be explored.

2. **(3)** In protein electrophoresis, proteins are electrically separated on a strip. It is a screening test to measure various proteins in body fluids, usually serum or urine. It assists in screening for diseases that are characterized by a increase or decrease in immunoglobulins. Complement fixation and antinuclear antibody testing are diagnostic studies for rheumatoid problems.

3. **(3)** The initial screening test for HIV is the ELISA. If the test is positive, confirmation of antibodies is done with a Western blot. Although serology and hepatitis screening along with a CBC and tuberculosis (TB) test are routinely performed, the initial work-up starts with an ELISA test. The CD4 count is performed during the active disease process.

4. **(1)** The majority of clients with systemic lupus erythematous have antinuclear antibodies in their blood. There is leukopenia, thrombocytopenia, lymphopenia, and a positive LE cell prep. Proteinuria with cellular casts is often noted.

5. **(4)** Angioedema is most easily seen in the eyes and mouth. It is edema of the mucous membrane tissue. It can also be observed on the tongue, feet, hands, and genitalia. Diffuse erythema may be seen in the upper body parts. Gastrointestinal symptoms, vomiting, cramping, and diarrhea may also be seen.

6. **(3)** The HIV antibody develops between 6 and 12 weeks after exposure. Because of the variability of antibody development, it is recommended that the test be repeated in 6 months to confirm the findings.

7. **(1)** The most reliable test for the presence of the specific IgE antibody is the skin test. RAST is less sensitive than skin testing, and it is difficult to standardize and reproduce results. The smear for eosinophils and the CBC are not specific for IgE antibody.

8. **(1)** Nasal smear for eosinophils is a simple office procedure. Many clients who have uncomplicated allergic rhinitis have a normal serum IgE. Skin testing should be performed by allergy-trained providers only. RAST testing is higher in cost and lower in sensitivity.

9. **(3)** A positive PPD for an immunocompetent child is 15 mm. For a child who is HIV positive, immunocompromised, or exposed to

an active case of TB, the child is considered positive at 5 mm. If the child (<4 years of age) has a chronic disease or has been exposed to HIV-positive people or people born in a foreign country, the child is considered positive at 10 mm.

10. **(4)** It is important to give the mother as much hope as possible but still be realistic about the condition. There is no way to tell when or if the child will convert to active AIDS. Many infants seroconvert to HIV-negative status.

11. **(3)** Although all of the tests mentioned in the answers may be included in a complete physical examination, laboratory tests specific to the diagnosis of SLE include the ANA, ESR, and C-reactive protein. During flares the ESR and C-reactive protein are elevated. The ANA titer in a client with SLE is positive at a 1:80 ratio.

## Disorders

12. **(2)** Egg albumin is just one of many identified common antigens that may result in anaphylactic reaction. Others include vaccines, allergen extracts, sulfonamides, penicillins, hormones, legumes (especially peanuts), berries, nuts, seafoods, and venomous stings (bee, wasp, yellow jacket stings). Changes in weather and strong scents and odors are triggers that may precipitate an asthma attack, resulting in bronchospasm and wheezing.

13. **(1)** There is a severe, life-threatening reduction of helper T cells, along with an increase in suppressor T cells. The helper T cells help amplify or increase the production of antibody-forming cells from the B lymphocytes after an encounter with an antigen. Killer T cells are produced after mature helper T cells interact with an antigen. Suppressor T cells suppress the formation of antibody-forming cells from the B lymphocytes; when their numbers are increased, this has a detrimental effect on the immunity and ability of the HIV-positive client to make antibody-forming cells.

14. **(2)** HIV infection creates a chronic infectious state in the body that is

transmitted via blood or body fluids and transplacentally.

15. **(3)** Ethical response includes notification of all persons at risk.

16. **(4)** This child is presenting with 4 of the 11 criteria necessary for diagnosing SLE. There is no single test for SLE, but the presence of these characteristics plus lab results can differentiate the diagnosis.

17. **(2)** The signs and symptoms presented are classic for allergic rhinitis. Acute bronchitis would present with cough and yellow or green sputum production. An asthma exacerbation would present with wheezing, chest tightness, decreased forced vital capacity, and history of exposure to an allergen. Influenza presents with fever, chills, and general malaise.

18. **(2)** The butterfly rash is one of the characteristic symptoms of SLE.

19. **(1)** The release of histamine results in bronchospasm, vasodilatation, and vascular permeability leading to wheezing, increased mucous production in the lung, and edema of the airway.

20. **(2)** Psychological and physical stress can exacerbate SLE. A balanced diet helps to limit the side effects of some of the medications, while regular exercise helps to reduce arthralgia and myalgia. Barrier contraception is recommended for the female with SLE. Pregnancy is usually allowed during periods of remission.

21. **(2)** Unprotected oral sex with an HIV-positive person puts you at risk for exposure to the virus. Contact such as casual kissing or sharing a room or bathroom does not transmit the virus. The virus is transmitted in bodily fluids and secretions.

22. **(3)** Frequent sexually transmitted diseases would alert the nurse practitioner to the client's lack of protected sex and the possibility of multiple partners. Night sweats, malaise, fatigue, swollen glands, and diarrhea can be associated with many other illnesses.

23. **(4)** The HIV virus is a retrovirus. It contains an enzyme, reverse transcriptase, that copies RNA into DNA. When the virus binds to a CD4 receptor, it inserts its RNA and enzymes into the cell, where a copy of the virus's RNA is made and enters the nucleus of the cell. As the infected host cell reproduces, the HIV DNA is duplicated and passed on.

24. **(4)** Although any of the above-mentioned clinical symptoms can be present in clients with SLE, fever, weight loss, and arthritis and arthralgias occur most often. Butterfly rash of the face and lymphadenopathy occur less than 50% of the time. Pulmonary effusion, hepatomegaly, splenomegaly, and Raynaud's syndrome occur in less than a third of the cases.

25. **(3)** The massive release of mediators triggers a series of events in target organs. Prior sensitization to the antigen must have occurred to trigger an anaphylactic reaction. Anaphylaxis may result from injection of an antigen, ingested food or drugs, or inhaled antigens.

26. **(2)** The onset of acute GVHD occurs between 30 and 50 days post-BMT. It results from immunocompetent donor T lymphocytes attacking the host tissues.

27. **(3)** The signs and symptoms of GVHD include maculopapular rash, generalized erythroderma with desquamation, increased bilirubin, increased serum glutamic-oxaloacetic transaminase (SGOT) and/or increased alkaline phosphatase, abdominal cramping, and diarrhea. Infection is characterized by fever, mental status changes, and headaches. Decreased RBC, hematocrit, and hemoglobin and petechiae are signs of anemia. Fever, chills, and urticaria are indications of a reaction to white cells in the marrow.

28. **(4)** T lymphocytes are the white cells responsible for control of the immune response. In SLE, T suppressor cells are decreased and cell activity is inhibited. This results in hypergammaglobulinemia and B-cell proliferation.

29. **(2)** The T4 lymphocyte is known as the T helper cell. These cells are responsible for the proliferation of lymphocytes and macrophages causing activation of the immune cells in response to an antigen. The B lymphocytes are effector cells that mediate humoral responses by production of antibodies. The band neutrophil and segmented neutrophil are slightly mature and fully mature neutrophils, respectively. Neutrophils are the most abundant cells in the bone marrow and blood.

30. **(3)** Based on the history of an HIV-positive test and the symptoms presented, the client is at risk for development of *P. carinii* pneumonia. Further examination would include obtaining a chest radiograph and pulse oximetry to determine oxygen saturation. The lack of purplish lesions is considered in ruling out Kaposi's sarcoma. *Klebsiella* pneumonia is a nosocomial infection, not community acquired. Lymphoma in HIV usually occurs as non-Hodgkin's at a primary site in the brain.

31. **(2)** Severe malaise, pallor, stridor, and dyspnea are signs and symptoms associated with a severe anaphylactic reaction. Symptoms may occur immediately or up to 2 hours after exposure. Severe reactions require immediate intervention.

32. **(3)** IgG is the major antibody against viruses and bacterias and is the principle mediator of the secondary immune response requiring repeated response to the same antigen. There is no IgC antibody. IgA is the secretory immunoglobulin found in tears, saliva, and mucous secretions of the lung and GI tract. IgE mediates allergic reactions.

33. **(2)** A type I hypersensitivity reaction causes an immediate wheal-and-flare reaction. Contact dermatitis is seen in a type IV (delayed) reaction. Hematuria is seen in a type II reaction caused by the presence of performed circulating cytotoxic antibodies, such as in a blood transfusion reaction or autoimmune hemolytic anemia. High fever can be seen in the type III hypersensitivity reaction when large quantities of antigen–antibody complexes are released in the body.

34. **(2)** Sexually active teenagers are the fastest growing group of HIV-positive clients because of unprotected sexual activity. Immunocompromised clients and family are at no greater risk for developing HIV than

is any other group. Risk factors for the development of HIV include unprotected sexual contact with someone of unknown HIV status, multiple sexual partners, intravenous drug use, hemophilia, and blood transfusions received prior to 1985.

35. **(2)** Live virus vaccinations should not be given for at least 5 months after gammaglobulin (IgG) therapy.

36. **(3)** Conjunctivitis is the most common ophthalmologic problem associated with SLE, along with hemorrhagic lesions secondary to hypertension or vasculitis. AV nicking can be seen in the client with hypertension. Brushfield's spots (white specks scattered around the entire circumference of the iris) strongly suggest Down's syndrome.

37. **(1)** Children with allergic rhinitis should monitor the air quality and allergy index in their area. A surgical-type mask will not filter out small allergens. Remaining inside during allergy season is an unrealistic expectation and can lead to depression and isolation for the child. Children can enjoy playing outdoors providing they avoid or are careful about the types of plants and flowers they are around. For example, the child with an allergy to ragweed should avoid areas where daisies, dahlias, and chrysanthemums are growing.

38. **(2)** Latex allergy is a progressive disease that worsens with continual exposure. The symptoms range from contact dermatitis to anaphylaxis. Currently, latex allergy affects 17% of the health care workers and 39% of dental professionals. Latex allergy is an acquired immune response to the latex protein allergen. There is no vaccine, and the only defense is to avoid contact with latex.

39. **(2)** The typical allergic facies consists of allergic shiners, Dennie lines (extra wrinkles below the lower eyelids), and mouth breathing. Nasal polyps are uncommon in childhood allergic rhinitis. The nasal discharge with allergies is usually clear.

40. **(3)** Common sites for atopic dermatitis are the popliteal and anticubital fossae, face, neck, upper arms and back, and dorsa of the hands, feet, fingers, and toes.

## Pharmacology

41. **(4)** Procainamide (Pronestyl), hydralazine (Apresoline), and isoniazid have been shown to induce a lupus-like syndrome. Discontinuation of the medication results in disappearance of the clinical signs and symptoms. Antibiotics such as sulfonamides (Septra DS) and penicillin (Pen VK, Penicillin G) have been associated with anaphylactic reactions in some clients. Oral contraceptives may cause increased blood pressure and increase the risk for development of thromboemboli. NSAIDs such as Motrin have been associated with gastrointestinal upset and gastric pain, especially when taken on an empty stomach.

42. **(2)** Epinephrine would be the first-line drug to be injected for the treatment of the respiratory distress associated with an anaphylactic reaction. The dosage for epinephrine (1:1000 SQ) subcutaneous is 0.01 ml/kg for a child and is 0.3–0.5 ml for an adult. Benadryl's onset of action is not fast enough. Lidocaine would only topically treat the pain and not the respiratory problem. Anti-inflammatory medications would not be given initially, but possibly later if needed.

43. **(4)** Chloroquine phosphate is the standard drug used for malaria prophylaxis. The dosage is 5 mg/kg body weight. Doxycycline (Vibramycin) is often used to treat diarrhea associated with traveling to areas where diarrhea is common from drinking the water; it is also used to treat chlamydia and pelvic inflammatory disease. Rocephin is used in bacterial septicemia or problems of the respiratory and urinary tract. Ampicillin (Polycillin, Omnipen) is used to treat a variety of organisms and as prophylaxis for bacterial endocarditis.

44. **(1)** Unless there is a secondary bacterial infection, antibiotics are not indicated. Antihistamines and reduction of exposure to the allergen will help to reduce the symptoms. For continued control and stabilization of the mast cell, corticosteroids are indicated.

45. **(3)** Trimethoprim-sulfamethoxazole (Septra, Bactrim) is used to treat as well as prevent *P. carinii* pneumonia. Usually a 21-day course of the drug is indicated. It may take 7–10 days to see a clinical response. Fluconazole (Diflucan) and amphotericin B are antifungal drugs; acyclovir (Zovirax) is an antiviral used primarily to treat herpes simple virus types 1 and 2 and herpes zoster (shingles).

46. **(2)** The chronic use of topical nasal decongestants for >3 days can result in a rebound effect when discontinued. This will lead to increased nasal congestion, called rhinitis medicamentosa. The nasal congestion is the result of reflex vasodilatation. The condition may take as long as 2–3 weeks to resolve. Allergic rhinitis is not a self-limiting illness associated only with the spring and fall. Even though therapy is initiated, the client should be instructed to avoid exposure to the allergen as much as possible.

47. **(4)** The second-generation antihistamines do not cross the blood–brain barrier; therefore, they do not cause sedation and/or psychomotor dysfunction. There is little anticholinergic activity and less dry mouth and constipation. The cost of these antihistamines is 15–30 times greater than the first-generation antihistamines. The medications are rapidly absorbed within 1–2 hours of oral administration on an empty stomach.

48. **(1)** Sympathomimetics (adrenergics) cause vasoconstriction, reducing edema and secretions. Inhaled corticosteroids stabilize mast cells and block degranulation.

49. **(3)** Chromolyn sodium is used to stabilize the mast cell membrane to prevent release of histamine when the cell comes in contact with an antigen. It does not affect the amount of histamine released from the cell, antagonize the effects of histamine, or reduce antiemetic activity.

50. **(2)** An advantage of using loratadine (Claritin) is the once-a-day dosing, which helps with client compliance. The cost is greater than some of the other first-generation antihistamines. An antihistamine/decongestant compound (loratadine/pseudoephedrine) is available either as twice-a-day dosing (Claritin D) or in an extended-release formulation for once-a-day dosing (Claritin D 24 Hour).

51. **(4)** Medications such as antihistamines and corticosteroids are used to counter mediator release and block release of additional mediators. NSAIDs, antibiotics, and decongestants are not indicated in the treatment of anaphylaxis.

52. **(4)** Both Benadryl and Dimetane are antihistamines and could be prescribed. The Dimetane would have less central nervous system sedating effects than the Benadryl. Benylin is an antitussive and Robitussin is an expectorant.

53. **(3)** While Benadryl will help with the itching and can certainly be administered after the child's distress is relieved, the immediate concern is to prevent respiratory arrest from swelling of the mucosa of the throat. The usual dose of epinephrine for children is 0.01 ml/kg of the 1:1000 solution.

# Head, Eyes, Ears, Nose, & Throat (HEENT)

## Physical Examination & Diagnostic Tests

### Head

1. In examining the mouth of a school-age child, the practitioner notes that the central and lateral permanent incisors have surface pitting and are stained brown. This condition is most suggestive of:

    1. The mother taking tetracycline during pregnancy.
    2. Poor dental hygiene.
    3. Dental fluorosis.
    4. Going to bed with a bottle during infancy.

2. The nurse practitioner is examining lymph nodes in the neck. What is palpated in the anterior triangle of the neck?

    1. Posterior cervical chain.
    2. Anterior superficial chain.
    3. Periauricular lymph nodes.
    4. Supraclavicular lymph nodes.

### Eyes

3. When using an ophthalmoscope on a child, the nurse practitioner:

    1. Holds the ophthalmoscope in the right hand (uses right eye) while examining the client's left eye.
    2. Starts the examination with the lens set at zero.
    3. Begins in a position 1 inch from the eye to check the red light reflex.
    4. Examines the anterior chamber in a well-lighted room and asks the child to focus on an object.

4. The visual screening for a 4-year-old child is recorded as 20/40 in both eyes. The nurse practitioner should now:

   1. Have the child return in 1 month to have his vision rechecked.

   2. Refer the child to an ophthalmologist.

   3. Recheck his vision to make sure that the measurement is accurate.

   4. Record the findings as normal for age.

5. The nurse practitioner checking for strabismus would use which test?

   1. Cover–uncover test.

   2. Bruchner's test. *Red reflex*

   3. Ishihara's test. *color*

   4. Snellen's test. *for vision*

6. The nurse practitioner observes lid lag in a client with:

   1. Myasthenia gravis. *ptosis*

   2. Hyperthyroidism.

   3. Hordeolum.

   4. Chalazion. *infection*

7. The nurse practitioner is preparing to examine the eyes of a child. In order to examine the optic disc and retinal vessels, the nurse practitioner uses what aperture on the ophthalmoscope?

   1. Small aperture.

   2. Red-free filter.

   3. Slit.

   4. Grid.

8. When testing the eyes for the presence of a normal consensual response, the nurse practitioner will:

   1. Shine the light into the client's pupil and observe the rate of pupillary constriction.

   2. Direct the light into one pupil and observe for the constriction or response of the other pupil.

   3. Hold a card in front of one eye and have the client focus on a fixed object, remove

   the card, and observe movement of the newly uncovered eye.

   4. Ask the client to focus on an object, then direct a light source to the bridge of the nose while observing for symmetrical reflection in both eyes.

9. When examining the eyes, the practitioner determines that the pupils change in size when the client refocuses from a close object to a distant object. This is interpreted as:

   1. Normal visual accommodation.

   2. Extraocular motor nerves are intact.

   3. Consensual response is appropriate.

   4. Visual acuity is within normal limits.

10. During a preschool screening for visual acuity, the nurse practitioner would also assess for:

    1. Pupils that are equal and reactive.

    2. Intraocular pressure by tonometry.

    3. Diplopia.

    4. Strabismus.

11. A nurse practitioner who is examining a 6-month-old infant finds that the corneal light reflex is asymmetrical. The nurse practitioner should first:

    1. Immediately refer this child to an ophthalmologist.

    2. Wait until the next well-child exam to re-evaluate the child's eyes.

    3. Further evaluate at this time with the cover–uncover test. *for strabismus*

    4. Check the red reflex.

12. A nurse practitioner is performing prekindergarten vision exams. One 5-year-old child who knows the alphabet well scores 20/40 with his left eye, 20/30 with his right eye, and 20/35 with both eyes. The nurse practitioner would:

    1. Explain to the mother that this is normal for this age group.

    2. Re-examine the child in 3 months.

3. Re-examine the child now with the Allen cards.

4. Refer the child for a more comprehensive exam.

13. Before testing a 5-year-old child's vision, the nurse practitioner determines which testing method to use based on the child's ability to recognize the alphabet. The best way to determine if the child knows the alphabet is to:

1. Ask the child if he/she knows the alphabet.

2. Bring the child close to the eye chart and ask the child to name several letters.

3. Have the child recite the alphabet.

4. Ask the child's parent if he/she knows the alphabet.

## Ears

14. When examining the ears of a child, the nurse determines the tympanic membrane is gray and translucent. This is interpreted as:

1. Scarring present from previous infections.

2. Decreased circulation to the membrane.

3. Presence of serous fluid behind the membrane.

4. Normal characteristics of the ear.

15. The purpose of conducting the Rinne test is to determine conduction of sound through the bone and through the auditory canal. A normal Rinne test is described as:

1. Equal conduction through the mastoid bone and the ear canal.

2. Air conduction twice as long as bone conduction.

3. Bone conduction twice as long as air conduction.

4. Sound is clearer with bone conduction than air conduction.

16. When assessing the tympanic membrane, specific landmarks are determined and described according to the face of a clock.

Where are normal landmarks for the right tympanic membrane located?

1. Direct light reflex at 5- to 6-o'clock position, malleus at 1- to 2-o'clock position, with umbo in center.

2. Manubrium slanted to the left with malleus at 10-o'clock position.

3. Direct light reflex in center of membrane with malleus at 9-o'clock position.

4. Umbo to the left with anterior malleolar folds at 10-o'clock position.

17. A 4-year-old's pure tone audiometry reveals 25 dB in the left ear and 43 dB in the right ear. The nurse practitioner would interpret these findings as:

1. Inconclusive because a pure tone audiometry is not accurate under age 5.

2. Within normal limits for age.

3. Normal hearing in the left ear and moderate hearing loss in the right ear.

4. Mild hearing loss in the left ear and normal hearing in the right ear.

18. The nurse practitioner knows that, if an infant has low or obliquely set ears, there is also an increased incidence of:

1. Cataracts.

2. Mental retardation.

3. Genitourinary defects.

4. Cardiovascular anomalies.

19. The National Institutes of Health (NIH) 1993 Consensus Statement on Early Identification of Hearing Impairment in Infants and Young Children recommends that auditory screening be implemented for:

1. All infants, preferably before discharge from the hospital nursery.

2. All premature infants, regardless of health status, by 6 months of age.

3. Only infants who have received ototoxic drug therapy, within 1 week of therapy.

4. All infants who have familial risk factors for hearing loss, by 3 months of age.

20. Tympanometry is used in the diagnosis of otitis media to determine:

    1. If the child has chronic hearing loss.

    2. Tympanic membrane compliance.

    3. The agent causing the otitis media.

    4. Which antibiotic to prescribe.

### Nose

21. The nurse practitioner understands that nasal mucosa:

    1. Is redder than oral mucosa.

    2. Is pale and translucent in appearance.

    3. Appears pink, boggy, without exudate.

    4. Appears dark pink with watery secretion.

### Throat

22. Throat cultures are indicated for which of the following suspects of pharyngitis?

    1. Rhinovirus and coronavirus viral infection.

    2. Group A β-hemolytic streptococci.

    3. Mononucleosis.

    4. *Candida albicans*.

23. The following statement is true regarding tonsils:

    1. Large tonsils in children are more prone to tonsillitis than small tonsils.

    2. Tonsils enlarge as the child grows older.

    3. Most hypertrophied tonsils in children are normal.

    4. The majority of tonsillitis is due to a β-hemolytic streptococcus infection.

24. An adolescent arrives at the nurse practitioner's clinic with a complaint of low-grade fever, sore throat, a slight headache, and fatigue. On physical examination, the nurse practitioner found exudative tonsils bilaterally, red pharynx with white patches, and enlarged posterior cervical neck nodes. The nurse practitioner would expect to find:

    1. Positive rapid strep test.

    2. Positive monospot test.

    3. Decreased white blood cell (WBC) count.

    4. Positive viral throat cultures.

## Disorders

### Head

25. An adolescent client presents to the nurse practitioner's office with a white plaque near the base of the tongue. The nurse practitioner notes that the plaque does not wipe off and assesses it as:

    1. Hemangioma.

    2. Hairy leukoplakia.

    3. Papilloma.

    4. Erythroplasia.

26. A adolescent client is being evaluated for a complaint of a sore throat. He states that he has difficulty swallowing and has some mouth pain. On exam, the nurse practitioner finds that the client's mouth, tongue, and pharynx are coated with white curd-like plaques that are difficult to remove with a tongue blade. The course of treatment for this client should include:

    1. Referral to an ear, nose, and throat (ENT) specialist.

    2. Amoxicillin 500 mg PO tid × 10 days.

    3. Encourage the client to have human immunodeficiency virus (HIV) screening.

    4. Clear liquids only for the next few days.

27. A 7-year-old is complaining of headaches. What physical assessment finding would cause the most concern?

    1. Pain is bilateral and described as tight or "bandlike."

    2. Headache consistently interrupts sleep at night.

    3. Headache is associated with intake of specific types of food.

    4. Pain is throbbing and localized in the occipital area.

28. The nurse practitioner taking a history on a preschooler learns that the family does not have fluoridated drinking water. Taking into consideration the concerns about fluorosis, the most appropriate nursing intervention would be to:

    1. Prescribe 5 ml of 0.2% fluoride solution (Fluorinse) once daily.
    2. Instruct parents to use a pea-size fluoridated dentifrice and to supervise toothbrushing.
    3. Instruct parents to use bottled drinking water.
    4. Refer to dentist for topical application of fluoride.

## Eyes

29. A mother reports that her toddler awoke this morning with redness and swelling of the eyelid. The nurse practitioner notes that the child is afebrile and the eyelid is nontender and is uniformly swollen. The most likely diagnosis is:

    1. Blepharitis.
    2. Hordeolum.
    3. Insect bite.
    4. Dacryocystitis.

30. Upon examination of a 2-week old infant, the nurse practitioner notes that the infant's left eye is watering and there is crusted material on the eyelids. No edema or erythema is noted. The nurse practitioner would make the diagnosis of:

    1. Nasolacrimal duct obstruction.
    2. Conjunctivitis.
    3. Congenital dacrocystocele.
    4. Corneal abrasion.

31. A 6-week-old infant is brought to the clinic by her mother. The mother is very concerned that the child's eyes are crossed. The best action for the nurse practitioner is:

    1. Explain to the mother this is not abnormal, and the child should be re-evaluated at 3 months of age.
    2. Refer the infant to an ophthalmologist.
    3. Provide the mother with normal saline eye drops for the infant.
    4. Have the mother alternate patching one eye, then the other, every 6 hours.

32. In assessing a child with bacterial conjunctivitis, the nurse practitioner finds:

    1. Minimal tearing, moderate itching, and profuse exudate.
    2. Severe itching, moderate tearing, and minimal discharge.
    3. Minimal itching, moderate tearing, and mucoid exudate.
    4. Minimal itching, moderate tearing, and profuse exudate.

33. The nurse practitioner makes the diagnosis of nasolacrimal obstruction in a 1-week-old infant who presents with "laking" of the right eye and a yellow discharge in the inner canthus of both eyes. Which of the following interventions would be contraindicated?

    1. Neosporin ophthalmic gtts.
    2. Massaging the lacrimal duct for 1 minute qid.
    3. Cleansing the eye with warm water qid.
    4. Dexamethasone (Decadron) ophthalmic gtts.

34. A 2-month-old infant presents to the nurse practitioner's office with an acutely red, tearing right eye. The rest of the physical exam is negative. The child's mother does not know what happened to the child's eye, but noted that the symptoms appeared after the baby awoke crying from a nap. There are no other children in the family and no indications to suspect unexplained trauma. Upon fluorescein exam, the nurse practitioner notes that there is green staining of the corneal epithelium and determines that the baby has:

    1. Corneal abrasion.
    2. Allergic conjunctivitis.
    3. Early periorbital cellulitis.
    4. Dacryocystitis.

35. At a 2-week well-child exam, the nurse practitioner notes that the infant has semipurulent discharge from the left eye. The mother reports that the eye has always been "watery" but has just gotten "gunky" in the last day or so. The prenatal and birth history is unremarkable. The nurse practitioner determines that the baby has a blocked tear duct and explains to the mother that, while this condition is very common, she wants to prescribe an antibiotic eye ointment for the mother to apply, in addition to tear duct massage qid, which the nurse practitioner demonstrates to her. The nurse practitioner prescribes erythromycin ophthalmic ointment because:

    1. It is less expensive than other medications and this family does not have insurance.

    2. It is important to cover the possibility of a chlamydia infection.

    3. The baby is too young for penicillin-based eye drops.

    4. The baby is too young for sulfa-based eye drops.

36. Bleeding into the anterior chamber of the eye, usually as a result of blunt trauma, results in a condition known as:

    1. Glaucoma.

    2. Chemical conjunctivitis.

    3. Hyphema.

    4. Corneal abrasion.

### Ears

37. A child is diagnosed by the nurse practitioner with acute otitis media. During pneumatic otoscopy, the nurse practitioner expects the tympanic membrane to be:

    1. Immobile, painful, with absent or decreased landmarks.

    2. Mobile, painful, with absent or decreased landmarks.

    3. Immobile, not painful, with landmarks visualized.

    4. Mobile, not painful, full, bulging.

38. A 6-year-old child is seen by the nurse practitioner for ear pain. The child is afebrile. The left ear canal is markedly edematous and moderately inflamed with thick, yellowish drainage at the external meatus. The child denies putting anything in the ear canal, but the nurse practitioner finds the child swims frequently. The most likely diagnosis is:

    1. Acute otitis media.

    2. Serous otitis media.

    3. Sinusitis.

    4. Otitis externa.

39. Which of the following organisms is least likely to cause otitis media?

    1. *Moraxella catarrhalis.*

    2. *Streptococcus pneumoniae.*

    3. *Chlamydia trachomatis.*

    4. *Haemophilus influenzae.*

40. Risk factors for acute otitis media include:

    1. Second-hand smoke, attending day care, American Indian and Eskimo race.

    2. Chinese race, previous otitis media, many siblings.

    3. Higher socioeconomic level, full-time day care, allergies.

    4. Summer season, full-time day care, premature at birth.

41. A 6-year-old child is examined by the nurse practitioner because of fluctuating hearing problems. The child is afebrile and denies otalgia. The mobility of the tympanic membrane is decreased when the nurse practitioner performs pneumatic otoscopy. The tympanic membrane is opaque with no visible landmarks. The child denies putting anything in the ear, and the mother states the child does not swim frequently. The most likely diagnosis is:

    1. Acute otitis media (AOM).

    2. A foreign body.

    3. Otitis media with effusion (OME).

    4. Otitis externa.

42. A 6-year-old girl is diagnosed by the nurse practitioner as having otitis externa. Appropriate treatment for otitis externa includes:

    1. Oral antibiotics, fever control, comfort measures, avoid exposure to sick people.

    2. Antibiotic/steroid otic drops, analgesia, avoidance of moisture in ears.

    3. Comfort measures, oral decongestants, antihistamines.

    4. No treatment is needed as the condition is self-limiting.

43. A 9-month-old infant has had six documented ear infections in the last 6 months. He lives in an environment with smokers, goes to day care, and is put to bed with a bottle so that his crying will not prevent his father, who gets up at 4 AM to go to work, from sleeping. You have spoken often with the mother regarding the risk factors for otitis media and the need to avoid smoke exposure for this infant. The mother does not seem to care; she refuses to think about quitting smoking and refuses to stop giving the child a bottle in bed. Day care is a necessity, due to the need for child care while the parents work. You are writing a prescription for the seventh ear infection. You should also consider:

    1. Calling Child Protective Services (CPS) to report the mother's noncaring attitude.

    2. Referring this child to a different primary care provider, who may develop a better rapport with the mother.

    3. Referring this child to an ENT physician for evaluation.

    4. Requesting a social service consult to assist with seeking different child care.

### Nose

44. An adolescent presents to the nurse practitioner's office with fever and complaints of right facial pain, copious yellow nasal discharge, and acute pain and headache when bending over for 5 days. There is no transillumination of the right maxillary sinus and that area is very tender to palpation. The adolescent diagnosis is:

    1. Chronic sinusitis.

    2. Acute sinusitis.

    3. Dental abscess.

    4. Common cold.

45. The nurse practitioner teaches the mother of a school-age child the following as the most effective preventive measure against the common cold:

    1. Judicious use of vitamin C during cold season.

    2. Ensuring adequate sleep and fluids.

    3. Meticulous handwashing, preferably with an antibacterial soap.

    4. Avoiding contact with children and adults who have a runny nose, cough, and sore throat.

46. A 4-year-old child has had an upper respiratory infection for 2 weeks with low-grade fever off and on. The child complains of cough during the daytime as well as at night. The child has bad breath, according to his mother, in spite of routine oral hygiene. He also has a runny nose with purulent discharge and is somewhat "crabby" as described by his mother. On physical exam, there are no ear infections, pharyngitis, or enlarged lymph nodes noted. This child most likely has:

    1. Streptococcal pharyngitis.

    2. A viral syndrome.

    3. Sinusitis.

    4. Infectious mononucleosis.

47. The nurse practitioner knows that the most common serious complication of sinusitis is:

    1. Orbital or periorbital cellulitis.

    2. Otitis media.

    3. Streptococcal pharyngitis.

    4. Infectious mononucleosis.

### *Throat*

48. An adolescent presents to the nurse practitioner's office with a chief complaint of "severe sore throat" for 3 days. The client states he also ran a fever but does not know how high it got, and he has been very tired with the sore throat. The physical exam revealed enlarged tonsils with large patchy exudate, inflamed pharynx, and nontender posterior cervical lymphadenopathy. The rest of the physical exam was nonremarkable. The nurse practitioner would make the diagnosis of:

    1. Infectious mononucleosis.

    2. Leukemia.

    3. Scarlet fever.

    4. Oral candidiasis.

49. Which of the following clinical findings are associated with bacterial streptococcal pharyngitis?

    1. Rhinorrhea.

    2. Cough.

    3. Enlarged tonsils with exudate.

    4. Small oral vesicles.

50. A 7-year-old presents to the nurse practitioner's office accompanied by his mother, who reports that the school sent home a note stating that strep throat is going around all classrooms. This child is not sick, but the mother wants him checked because he frequently gets strep throat. After a thorough physical exam, including a rapid throat culture, with negative findings, the nurse practitioner tells this mother that the child is not ill and reviews with her the signs and symptoms of illness and when she should call or return to the office for further care or advice. This mother insists that she wants a prescription to prevent him from getting strep throat, since he is so susceptible and they have a vacation planned in 2 days and she does not want him to be sick for that. The nurse practitioner would:

    1. Prescribe a full 10-day course of antibiotic because the mother is insistent.

    2. Explain to the mother that antibiotics do not necessarily protect from future illness.

    3. Prescribe an abbreviated 3-day course of antibiotics and tell the mother that this is prophylactic therapy.

    4. Refer her to your collaborating physician, because you know he will prescribe antibiotics for her child.

51. The nurse practitioner treats a 10-year-old female for documented pharyngitis caused by group A β-hemolytic streptococcus infection. The child's mother calls the nurse practitioner at 10 PM after 12 hours of antibiotic therapy to tell you that the child has a rash and she is not sure if she should continue the antibiotic. Upon questioning, the nurse practitioner determines that the rash is on the trunk, is very red, and feels rough like sandpaper. It does not itch and does not look like hives. The child is not having any facial swelling or difficulty breathing. The nurse practitioner tells the mother:

    1. To discontinue the antibiotic immediately, as this is likely an allergic reaction.

    2. To take the child to the emergency room to be evaluated.

    3. That this is most likely a strep rash, which can still appear after initiation of therapy.

    4. That this rash is probably a viral exanthem, and not related to the strep throat.

## Pharmacology

52. The antibiotic(s) of choice for acute sinusitis in the adolescent is(are):

    1. Amoxicillin (Amoxil) 500 mg tid PO × 14 days; trimethoprim-sulfamethoxazole (Bactrim) DS 1 q12h PO × 14 days, Penicillin V-K (Pen Vee K) 500 mg bid PO × 14 days.

    2. Trimethoprim-sulfamethoxazole DS 1 q12h PO × 14 days, Penicillin V-K (Pen Vee K) 500 mg bid PO × 14 days.

3. Penicillin G 150,000 U IM × 1; amoxicillin 500 mg tid PO × 14 days.

4. Amoxicillin 500 mg tid PO × 14 days; trimethoprim-sulfamethoxazole DS 1 q12h PO × 14 days.

53. Which antibiotic would be appropriate for the nurse practitioner to prescribe for β-lactamase production by strains of *Haemophilus influenzae* and *Moraxella catarrhalis* in a child with acute otitis media?

   1. Amoxicillin (Amoxil).

   2. Trimethoprim-sulfamethoxazole (Bactrim).

   3. Penicillin V-K.

   4. Metronidazole (Flagyl).

54. Prophylactic antibiotics are indicated for which of the following clients?

   1. A 3-year-old with two episodes of AOM in the previous winter.

   2. A 2-year-old with three episodes of AOM within the last 6 months.

   3. A 4-year-old with history of prophylactic antibiotics in the last 2 years but without evidence of AOM this year.

   4. A 2-year-old with three episodes of AOM over the last 9 months.

55. The treatment plan for an adolescent diagnosed with infectious mononucleosis includes which of the following?

   1. Bed rest during acute phase.

   2. Avoid exercise during acute phase.

   3. Corticosteroids during acute phase.

   4. Ampicillin orally for 10 days.

56. An adolescent client has had yellowish green nasal drainage and frontal headache for a week. The adolescent's temperature has gone up to 101.2°F on most afternoons and she has a cough that worsens when she lies down. The physical exam is within normal limits except for the drainage and a slightly erythematous pharynx. She does not have any drug allergies and has not been on any medications in the last few months. Which medication would be best to prescribe for her?

   1. Diphenhydramine hydrochloride (Benadryl).

   2. Erythromycin (E-Mycin).

   3. Pseudoephedrine hydrochloride (Sudafed).

   4. Amoxicillin (Amoxil).

57. A toddler (weight 18 kg) is diagnosed as having bilateral otitis media. His last ear infection was 6 months ago and he has no known drug allergies. An appropriate medication to prescribe would be:

   1. Ampicillin, 125 mg/kg, 1 tsp tid PO × 7 days.

   2. Corticosteroid otic solution, 3 gtts both ears × 10 days.

   3. Amoxicillin, 250 mg/kg, 1 tsp tid PO × 10 days.

   4. Doxycycline 250 mg, 1 tsp tid PO × 10 days.

58. An infant's mother calls the nurse practitioner's office to report that her son has white patches on the insides of his cheeks and on his tongue. The baby is 2 months old and is breast-fed. He is feeding okay today, but not quite as well as usual. The mother thinks he acts like his mouth hurts when he sucks. The nurse practitioner determines that the baby has oral thrush and tells the mother that she will call in a prescription for some medication. The nurse practitioner also instructs the mother that the best way to give the medication is to:

   1. Use a Q-Tip to paint the white patches with the medicine qid after the baby eats.

   2. Squirt a dropperful of the medication into the baby's mouth three times a day before she feeds him.

   3. Rotate the baby's head from side to side to equally distribute the medication around the baby's mouth.

   4. Squirt a dropperful of the medication into the baby's mouth qid after she feeds him.

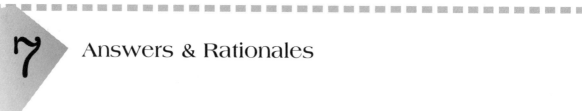

# Answers & Rationales

## Physical Examination & Diagnostic Tests

### Head

1. **(3)** Dental fluorosis causes surface pitting and staining, especially to the central and lateral permanent incisors. Tetracycline would have caused staining of all the teeth. Dental caries would be more indicative of poor dental hygiene. "Baby teeth," not the permanent teeth, would be affected by going to bed with a bottle.

2. **(2)** The conceptualization of triangles is useful in determining the location of palpable lymph nodes in the neck. The sternocleidomastoid muscle is the division between the anterior (containing the anterior superficial cervical chain) and the posterior (containing the posterior cervical chain) triangles. The trapezius muscle marks the posterior border of the posterior triangle. The supraclavicular or scale nodes are palpated in the angle formed by the clavicle and the sternocleidomastoid muscle.

### Eyes

3. **(2)** The correct use of the ophthalmoscope involves using the right hand and right eye to examine the client's right eye. The room should be semidarkened for best visualization. The examiner initially inspects the lens and vitreous body from a distance of about 12 inches (at zero setting) and moves closer to the eye, usually rotating the lenses to the positive numbers (+15 to +20), which assists in focusing on near objects.

4. **(4)** A 4-year-old's normal acuity is 20/40; therefore, none of the other answers is appropriate.

5. **(1)** Cover–uncover tests for strabismus; Bruchner's tests the red reflex, Ishihara's tests color perception, and Snellen's tests far vision.

6. **(2)** If the lid margin falls above the limbus (junction line where the sclera and cornea meet) so that some sclera is visible, hyperthyroidism may be present. The lid may lag behind the limbus as the gaze moves from an upward to a downward position. Ptosis is a drooping lid margin that falls at the pupil or below and may indicate and oculomotor lesion or myasthenia gravis. A chalazion is an inflammation or cyst of the meibomian glands that lie within the posterior portion of the eyelid. A localized infection of the small glands around the eyelashes in the hair follicle at the lid margin is called a hordeolum.

7. **(2)** The red-free filter is used to examine the optic disc for pallor and vascular changes as well as to assess for retinal hemorrhages. The small aperture is used for small pupils, the slit is for the anterior eye, and the grid for estimating the size of lesions found in the fundal area.

8. **(2)** Consensual response is pupillary constriction of one eye when there is a direct light stimulus to the pupil of the other eye.

9. **(1)** Changes in pupil size when refocusing from near to distant objects is normal accommodation. Extraocular eye movements (EOMs) refer to the ability to move the eye. Consensual response is constriction of the eye in response to light being shined in the opposite eye. The Snellen eye chart is used to determine the visual acuity.

10. **(4)** Strabismus (malalignment of the eyes) can be a precursor for amblyopia (decreased visual acuity). It is important to detect strabismus as early as possible in preschool children. Options #1 and #3 are components of a neurologic assessment. Tonometry exams are performed to assess for glaucoma.

11. **(3)** While the corneal light reflection test is a quick screening test for strabismus, the cover–uncover test is more sensitive in determining the presence of strabismus.

12. **(4)** It is standard to refer children with a one-line discrepancy between eyes. It would also be helpful to ask the mother if she has concerns about the child's vision.

13. **(2)** Parents and children may misrepresent their ability to recognize letters of the alphabet. Being able to recite the alphabet is not indicative of ability to recognize letters. Bringing the child close to the chart and asking him to identify letters assures the ability without risking error due to far vision deficits.

## Ears

14. **(4)** This describes the normal characteristics of the tympanic membrane. There is no evidence of scarring or fluid.

15. **(2)** The normal Rinne test is air conduction twice as long as bone conduction.

16. **(1)** This describes the correct position for these landmarks on the right ear. In Option #2, the manubrium slants to the right with the malleus at the 1- to 2-o'clock position for the right ear. Option #3 describes the correct position for the left ear. In Option #4, the umbo is in the center with the anterior folds at the 1- to 2-'o'clock position for the right ear.

17. **(3)** Pure tone audiometry is appropriate after age 3; 0–25 dB is normal, 26–40 dB is mild hearing loss, and 41–55 dB is moderate hearing loss.

18. **(3)** Low-set or obliquely set ears occur more frequently in children who also have genitourinary defects. None of the other defects is associated with low-set ears.

19. **(1)** The NIH 1993 Consensus Statement on Early Identification of Hearing Impairment in Infants and Young Children recommends that auditory screening be implemented for all infants, of both high and low risk, within the first 3 months of life but preferably before discharge from the hospital nursery. The panel emphasizes that comprehensive intervention and management for those infants identified with hearing loss must be an integral part of a universal screening program.

20. **(2)** Tympanometry is being used more frequently as an aid in the diagnosis of otitis media. It gives an estimate of tympanic membrane compliance. Compliance may be normal early in the infection, but compliance will decrease as the fluid increases in the middle ear.

## Nose

21. **(1)** Nasal mucosa is redder than oral mucosa. Increased redness of the nasal mucosa usually indicates infection. Pale, boggy turbinates along with watery secretion often occurs with allergic rhinitis. The normal secretion is mucoid. Purulent, crusty, or bloody secretions are abnormal.

## Throat

22. **(2)** Rapid screening for strep can be done from a throat swab with antigen agglutination kits, but there is a 5–10% false-negative rate; therefore, it is suggested that culture should be performed. The sensitivity and specificity (95% specific and 90% sensitive) of the heterophile antibody test (monospot test), which rapidly detects heterophile antibodies, compare with those of older heterophile antibody tests to diagnose mononucleosis. *Candida albicans* and rhinovirus are not diagnosed by bacterial cultures. Oral candidiasis can be diagnosed with a potassium hydroxide smear.

23. **(3)** Enlarged tonsils are common in young children. As the child grows older, the tonsils recede in size. Only about 25–30% of tonsillitis is caused by the β-hemolytic streptococcus. Option #1 is a false statement.

24. **(2)** The client in this situation had risk factors (age) and symptoms of mononucleosis; therefore, the monospot or heterophile antibody test should be conducted. The classic triad of mononucleosis symptoms is sore throat, fever, and posterior cervical lymphadenopathy with or without mild tenderness. Rapid screening for strep can be done from a throat swab with antigen agglutination kits and would be obtained first; however, it would probably be negative. A WBC count would be ordered for bacterial pharyngitis, in the WBC elevation is found with bacterial infection and a decrease is associated with viral agents.

## Disorders

### Head

25. **(2)** Leukoplakia is a white patch present on the oral mucosa that cannot be rubbed off. Hemangiomas are benign blood vessel proliferation of the lips, tongue, or buccal mucosa. Erythroplasia is an asymptomatic, red, velvety lesion of the mouth. Papillomas are benign verrucous lesions that are manifestations of human papillomavirus infection.

26. **(3)** Adolescents who present with thrush (oral candidiasis) may be immunologically impaired. It is important to make the diagnosis of HIV early to start treatment modalities. Treatment with amoxicillin may actually worsen the condition.

27. **(2)** Headaches (HA) that arouse the child from sleep could be indicative of serious underlying problems. HA may also be associated with food, if so then the identified food should be avoided. Bilateral constricting throbbing HAs are more likely to be characteristic of chronic nonprogressive types, i.e., tension HA.

28. **(2)** A fluoridated dentifrice should be used in a small amount (pea-size), and children under 6 should be supervised so that they do not swallow too much toothpaste, which would put them at risk for fluorosis. The dose of fluoride rinse is too high, plus it is inappropriate to prescribe to a preschooler. Bottled water usually does not contain fluoride. Topical application, though appropriate, is not the best answer.

### Eyes

29. **(3)** Generalized, diffuse swelling and erythema of the eyelid is associated with an insect bite. Blepharitis is a chronic inflammatory condition characterized by erythema and scaling of the lid margins. Hordeolum, or stye, is a acute, purulent inflammation of the sebaceous glands (usually the meibomian or zeisian) of the eyelids and usually does not involve the entire eyelid. It may be painful, especially over the gland. Dacryocystitis is an inflammation of the lacrimal sac characterized by erythema and swelling over the lacrimal duct.

30. **(1)** Nasolacrimal obstruction occurs in up to 6% of infants. Signs and symptoms include a wet eye with mucoid discharge. There may also be irritated skin and conjunctivitis associated with this condition. There is no redness that would be indicative of conjunctivitis. Congenital dacrocystocele presents at birth as a bluish subcutaneous mass. There would be more signs of irritation and pain with a corneal abrasion.

31. **(1)** Strabismus is not an uncommon or abnormal occurrence in infants up until 3 months of age.

32. **(4)** Classic signs of bacterial conjunctivitis include those symptoms listed along with complaints of eyelids being "glued shut" upon arising in the morning. Option #2 is indicative of allergic conjunctivitis. Option #3 is indicative of viral conjunctivitis.

33. **(4)** Steroid (dexamethasone) medications are not used to treat nasolacrimal obstruction in infancy. Due to the yellow discharge in the eye, it would be appropriate to prescribe an antibiotic to prevent and/or treat conjunctivitis. Cleansing the eye with warm water and

massaging the lacrimal duct are both appropriate interventions.

34. **(1)** The baby is demonstrating signs of corneal abrasion, which is often inflicted by the baby's own fingernails. The fluorescein test is specific for abraded corneal epithelium. Allergic conjunctivitis would not present in this fashion. Periorbital cellulitis involves the tissues surrounding the eye and is associated with illness, often fever. Dacryocystitis (blocked tear duct) does not occur with a sudden onset at this age.

35. **(2)** Until the results of a culture of the drainage are obtained, the nurse practitioner should be aware of the possibility of chlamydia infection, which could have been contracted during a vaginal delivery.

36. **(3)** Treatment of hyphema requires initial stabilization, which includes patching and referral to an ophthalmologist for complete management. Chemical conjunctivitis is inflammation of the conjunctiva caused by exposure to a chemical irritant. Corneal abrasion is abrading of the corneal epithelium by contact with a foreign object.

### Ears

37. **(1)** The diagnosis of otitis media is clinical, made by otoscopy based on the appearance of the tympanic membrane. The bony landmarks are absent or decreased. The tympanic membrane may be full, bulging, or retracted with pus, and the light reflex is distorted. Pneumatic otoscopy reveals decreased or absent mobility of the tympanic membrane. Erythema is an inconclusive finding, especially in children, because the redness may be due to crying rather than infection.

38. **(4)** The child has the clinical findings of otitis externa. Otitis externa is an inflammation and/or infection of the external ear canal predisposed by excessive wetness, as in swimming. Common organisms responsible for otitis externa include *Pseudomonas aeruginosa*, *Proteus mirabilis*, and *Enterobacter aerogenes*. Sinusitis clinical findings focus on sinus tenderness and a purulent nasal discharge. Clinical findings of otitis media include ear pain, full or bulging tympanic membrane,

decreased or negative mobility, and possible erythema. Findings associated with serous otitis media include opaque or translucent tympanic membrane with presence of air bubbles; landmarks may be absent and the light reflex may be diffuse or absent.

39. **(3)** The key factor that contributes to acute otitis media (AOM) is a dysfunctional eustachian tube that may allow bacteria from the nasopharynx to the middle ear. The most frequent bacterial organisms that infect the middle ear, especially in children, are similar to those of the nasopharynx: *Streptococcus pneumoniae*, *Haemophilus influenzae*, and *Moraxella catarrhalis*. *Escherichia coli* and *Klebsiella* cause about 15% of AOM cases in babies under 6 weeks old. Viruses may also cause AOM. *Chlamydia trachomatis* is not a frequent causative agent.

40. **(1)** AOM occurs more during the fall, winter, and spring than summer. American Indians and Eskimos have more repetitive and severe otitis media than members of other races. Children who attend day care centers have more frequent infections than those who do not. Members of lower socioeconomic levels are more at risk than those at higher levels. Other risk factors are living with many siblings or in homes with smokers, developmental abnormalities, and male gender.

41. **(3)** The client with otitis externa, "swimmer's ear," or inflammation of the external auditory canal presents with ear pain. The most common clinical findings include redness and swelling of the external ear canal, pain with manipulation of movement of the auricle, and no swelling or pain over the mastoid; the tympanic membrane (TM) is not usually involved. The TM is involved in acute otitis media. There was no evidence in the case of the child placing a foreign body in the ear. The most significant distinction between otitis media with effusion and acute otitis media is that clinical findings of acute infection, such as fever and otalgia, are lacking in OME. OME is the most common cause of hearing loss in children. OME clinical findings include relatively asymptomatic, decreased mobility, and bulging opaque TM with no visible landmarks.

42. **(2)** Treatment goals for otitis externa include decreasing inflammation and combating infection in the auditory canal. Unless there is a concurrent otitis media or generalized illness with fever, or the local infection is severe, oral antibiotics are not needed. The child should be taught to keep the ear canals clean and dry and to not use Q-Tips, which can abrade the ear canal. Swimming should be avoided for 7–10 days. Showering should be done only with occlusive covers (i.e., cotton-balls coated with Vaseline).

43. **(3)** With the frequency and persistence of ear infections, this child is at risk for hearing loss secondary to middle ear effusions. He needs to be evaluated for the possibility of pneumatic equalization tube insertion to facilitate drainage. This mother's behavior is not neglectful, in CPS terms. Changing child care arrangements is unlikely to be helpful because of the passive smoke exposure in the child's home environment.

### Nose

44. **(2)** The adolescent is experiencing the classic characteristics of acute sinusitis. Chronic sinusitis has nasal discharge, congestion, headache, or cough for over 30 days. A dental abscess has a severe, tooth-associated pain and jaw tenderness.

45. **(3)** Transmission of cold viruses is spread indirectly (e.g., self-innoculation from virus being on surfaces of inanimate objects, to mucous membranes of the nose and mouth). It is less likely to be spread by aerosol method. So the child should avoid touching the nose and mouth unless the hands have been thoroughly washed. It is impractical to avoid contact as cold viruses are found everywhere. Although many individuals believe vitamin C prevents colds, there is little research to support the claim.

46. **(3)** The above-described symptoms are classic for sinusitis. Streptococcal pharyngitis is not usually associated with runny nose and upper respiratory symptoms, but rather with acute onset and high fever, headache, stomachache, and history of exposure to strep infection. Viral syndromes usually improve within 7–10 days. Infectious mononucleosis is a possibility to be considered when illnesses linger. Children with mono usually complain of sore throat and have enlarged lymph nodes and generalized malaise.

47. **(1)** While any of the above conditions may be associated with or follow sinusitis, orbital or periorbital cellulitis is the most common serious complication of sinusitis. The ethmoid sinus is separated from the orbit by the thin lamina papayracea. Erosion of this bone leads to invasion of the orbit by bacterial pathogens. The eyelids appear intensely red and swollen. Fever, malaise, and increased WBCs are present. Orbital pain, proptosis, and limitation of eye movement helps distinguish this condition from preseptal cellulitis. Treatment involves parenteral antibiotics and consultation with an ophthalmologist and otolaryngologist to determine whether surgical drainage is indicated.

### Throat

48. **(1)** Mononucleosis is commonly seen in adolescents and young adults. It often presents with fever, exudate on the tonsils, generalized lymphadenopathy, malaise, posterior cervical adenopathy and palatine petechiae. Leukemia presents with anorexia, irritability, lethargy, and bone pain. The peak incidence is in 3- to 5-year-olds. Scarlet fever presents in children 2–10 years old with fever, abdominal pain, headache, sore throat, and strawberry tongue. Oral candidiasis presents with white curd-like plaques on an erythematous mucosa. The tongue is red with a white coat.

49. **(3)** Characteristics of bacterial pharyngitis include headache, mild to severe erythema of the tonsils with white or yellow exudate, dysphagia, positive anterior cervical nodes, sore throat with dysphagia, fever >101°–102.5°, and nausea. Viral organisms that cause herpangina present with small oral vesicles. Cough is the primary symptom of acute bronchitis. Rhinorrhea is associated with allergic rhinitis.

50. **(2)** Explain to this mother that unnecessary antibiotic therapy, while not only not preventative, may be harmful to her child because of developing antibiotic resistance,

which may render antibiotics ineffective in the future due to inappropriate overuse.

51. **(3)** The described rash is classic for scarlet fever, which is an erythematous papular eruption, sometimes associated with generalized erythema, concentrated on the trunk and proximal extremities. It feels like fine sandpaper, and can occur within 1–4 days of the onset of the focal infection, such as pharyngitis, vaginitis, cellulitis, erythema of palms and soles, and strawberry tongue. The rash may desquamate in recovery phase. Allergic reactions to antibiotics are urticarial in nature and associated with itching and even respiratory difficulty in severe reactions.

## Pharmacology

52. **(4)** Amoxicillin (Amoxil) is the first-line antibiotic for acute uncomplicated sinusitis in the adolescent because of cost-effectiveness, efficacy, and cure rates ranging from 67% to 100%. Even though 35% of *H. influenzae* and 75% of *M. catarrhalis* produce β-lactamase, cure rates when using amoxicillin have not been significantly different. Therefore, several other drugs may be utilized with similar clinical response to amoxicillin. These include ampicillin, trimethoprim-sulfamethoxazole (Bactrim), cefaclor (Ceclor), cefuroxime axetil (Ceftin), loracarbef (Lorabid), and amoxicillin–clavulanate potassium (Augmentin).

53. **(2)** Amoxicillin is ineffective against β-lactamase production. Erythromycin-sulfisoxazole, trimethoprim-sulfamethoxazole, and cephalosporins are effective against β-lactamase production by strains of *H. influenzae* and *M. catarrhalis*. Penicillin V-K and metronidazole are not effective in this group. Cephalexin, cefuroxime, or cefixime can be used as alternatives.

54. **(2)** The decision to prescribe prophylactic antibiotics is individualized but should be considered for children who have experienced three documented episodes of acute otitis media in a 6-month period. This risks and benefits should be explained to the parents. Antibiotic prophylaxis has been found to be as effective as ventilating tubes in preventing new cases of AOM.

55. **(1)** The treatment of mononucleosis includes bed rest while the client has fever and myalgia (10–14 days), supportive acetaminophen or ibuprofen, warm saline gargles, and throat lozenges or spray. The client must avoid strenuous exercise and contact sports the first 2–3 weeks. Corticosteroids are recommended only in clients with impending airway obstruction. Ampicillin is not recommended due to allergic reaction and rash reaction. About 95% of clients with mononucleosis recover uneventfully with supportive treatment.

56. **(4)** The client is experiencing symptoms of acute sinusitis. The first-line antibiotic to prescribe for this condition is amoxicillin due to safety and efficacy. Oral antihistamines such as diphenhydramine should not be used unless the client has allergies. Oral decongestants (pseudoephedrine hydrochloride) are not as effective in clients with sinusitis as topical agents. Erythromycin is not a first-line antibiotic for sinusitis.

57. **(3)** The recommended treatment for otitis media in a toddler is amoxicillin 40 mg/kg/day or, for this child, 250 mg, 1 tsp tid for 10 days. In a child under 20 kg the recommendation is ampicillin 50–100 mg/kg/day or, for this child, 250 mg, 1 tsp qid for 10 days. Erythromycin or trimethoprim-sulfamethoxazole (Bactrim) are other alternatives.

58. **(1)** Using a Q-Tip to apply the medication directly to the plaques ensures better coverage than squirting the medication into the baby's mouth. Giving the medication after feedings allows prolonged contact with the plaques prior to the next bathing of the oral mucosa with formula or breast milk. Be sure to remind the mother to use a new Q-Tip each time she puts one into the medication bottle, as going from the mouth to the bottle with the same Q-Tip can contaminate the medication remaining in the bottle.

# Integumentary & Childhood Diseases

**8**

## Physical Examination & Diagnostic Tests

1. The nurse practitioner describes an annular skin lesion as usually arranged in:

   1. Groups of vesicles erupting unilaterally.

   2. A line.

   3. A pattern of merging together, not discrete.

   4. A circle or ring.

2. The nurse practitioner is inspecting a dark-skinned child for signs of jaundice. The best place to observe is:

   1. Sclera of the opened eye.

   2. Palms of the hands and soles of the feet.

   3. Oral mucosa.

   4. Nail beds.

3. The Wood's lamp is used to evaluate skin lesions. When the light is shined on the client's skin, a green–yellow fluorescence indicates:

   1. Presence of fungi.

   2. Lichenification.

   3. Keratinized cells.

   4. Bacterial colonies.

4. On examination of a client's skin, the nurse practitioner finds a lesion that is about 0.75 cm in diameter, brown, circumscribed, flat, and nonpalpable. The correct term for this lesion is:

   1. Macule.

   2. Papule.

   3. Nodule.

   4. Wheal.

5. The history and physical of a client indicates past occurrences of lichenification. The nurse practitioner identifies the characteristics of this lesion as:

   1. Dried, crusty exudate, slightly elevated.

   2. Rough, thickened epidermis; accentuated skin markings.

   3. Keratinized cells shaped in an irregular pattern with exfoliation.

   4. Loss of epidermis with hollowed-out area and dermis exposed.

6. Clubbing of the nails occurs in clients with chronic respiratory conditions. The nurse practitioner assesses for this condition by:

   1. Evaluating the nail for transverse depressions and ridges.

   2. Placing both of the client's hands together with palms inward and index fingers aligned.

   3. Placing nail beds of each index finger together to determine angle of nail plate.

   4. Determining if these is diffuse discoloration of the nail bed from decreased oxygenation.

7. A circumscribed, elevated lesion >1 cm in diameter and containing clear serous fluid is best described as a:

   1. Papule.

   2. Vesicle.

   3. Bulla.

   4. Pustule.

8. In performing a skin assessment, the nurse practitioner understands that the following characteristic of a mole would necessitate immediate intervention:

   1. A 5-mm, symmetric, uniformly brown mole on the thigh that has been present and has not changed in appearance for over 5 years.

   2. Multiple small (1- to 3-mm) flat moles across the upper back that are dark brown in color, round, and have smooth edges.

   3. A 3-cm waxy papule, with a "stuck-on" appearance, noted on the face.

   4. A new 2-mm mole that is brown with a red, irregular border, and is occasionally pruritic.

9. Dermatophyte skin infections can be diagnosed from skin scrapings and prepped with which solution for microscopic exam?

   1. Hydrochloric acid.

   2. 20% potassium hydroxide (KOH) solution.

   3. Gram's stain.

   4. Distilled water.

10. When administering skin tests to an immunocompromised client, the nurse practitioner must consider:

    1. The importance of not applying more than one skin test at a time.

    2. That the skin test may react more aggressively than expected.

    3. Identifying a known allergen for the client and utilizing it as a control.

    4. That the immunocompromised client should not be skin tested.

11. The nurse is examining a 6-week-old infant of Latin American descent. There are irregular areas of deep blue pigmentation across the infant's buttocks. The nurse would identify this as characteristic of:

    1. Child abuse.

    2. Telangiectatic nevi.

    3. Cutis marmorata.

    4. Mongolian spots.

# Skin Disorders

12. An adolescent client complains of intolerable itching in the pubic hair. On examination, the nurse practitioner notes erythematous papules and tiny white specks in the pubic hair. The differential diagnosis includes all **except**:

    1. Pediculosis pubis.

    2. Scabies.

3. Impetigo.

3. Atopic dermatitis.

13. An adolescent girl has an area of vesicles in clusters with an erythematous base that extend from her spine, around and under her arm and breast to the sternum on her left side. She says the area was very "sore" last week and the vesicles started erupting yesterday. She is complaining of severe pain in the area. The diagnosis for this conditions is:

1. Psoriasis.

2. Herpes zoster.

3. Contact dermatitis.

4. Cellulitis.

14. A chronic skin condition sometimes associated with arthritis is:

1. Eczema.

2. Psoriasis.

3. Neurodermatitis.

4. Pityriasis rosea.

15. Which is a true statement about psoriasis?

1. It usually is worse in the summer.

2. It is highly contagious.

3. It can be aggravated by stress.

4. All clients have accompanying pruritis.

16. A mother brings her school-age child in for examination. She reports the child has been noted to be frequently scratching and the itching seems to be worse at night. Upon examination, the nurse practitioner notes lesion on the sides of the fingers and inner aspect of the elbows. These lesions are short, irregular runs approximately 2–3 mm long and the width of a hair. The nurse practitioner tells the mother she suspects:

1. Scabies.

2. Hives.

3. Fleas.

4. Ticks.

17. The following are all true statements regarding urticaria **except** for:

1. Most cases of acute urticaria are mediated by immunoglobulin E mast cell degranulation after exposure to certain substances.

2. Chronic urticaria may be related to occult infections.

3. Urticaria is characterized by itchy red swellings of a few millimeters to a few centimeters in size.

4. Laboratory studies are necessary to identify the causative agent.

18. An adolescent client who is known to be human immunodeficiency virus (HIV) positive presents with several painless, persistent, raised purple lesions on the face. The most likely cause is:

1. Seborrheic dermatitis.

2. Molluscum contagiosum.

3. Kaposi's sarcoma.

4. Fungal infection.

19. In making a differential diagnosis between nummular eczema (dermatitis) and dyshidrotic eczematous dermatitis, the nurse practitioner knows:

1. Nummular eczema is characterized by flushing and clusters of papulopustules on the cheek and forehead.

2. Dyshidrotic eczematous dermatitis is a chronic vesicular type of hand and foot eczema characterized by vesicles (tapioca-like), scaling, lichenification, and pruritius.

3. Nummular eczema is a hereditary disorder characterized by chronic scaling plaques that are usually appear bilaterally on exposed areas (knees, elbows).

4. Dyshidrotic eczematous dermatitis affects primarily young adults, is contagious, and is characterized by firm papules with a clefted surface and multiple conical vegetations.

20. An 11-year-old male client presents to the clinic with a complaint of being bitten last night by another child during a fight. He has a deep bite mark on his forearm and the skin has been broken. His records indicate that he has had a tetanus shot about 8 years ago. Recommended treatment by the family nurse practitioner should include all **except**:

    1. Administer 0.5 ml of tetanus toxoid IM.

    2. Instruct client to watch for signs of infection.

    3. Initiate treatment with penicillin plus a penicillinase-resistent penicillin.

    4. Close wound with sutures or Steri-strips.

21. Nail involvement secondary to primary foot and hand tinea that is characterized by accumulation of subungual keratin that produces thickened, distorted, crumbling nails is termed:

    1. Hippocratic nails.

    2. Onychomycosis.

    3. Koilonychia.

    4. Anonychia.

22. An adolescent boy presents for an office visit with complaint of a measles-like rash on his trunk and spreading to the extremities. He was seen several days ago for bronchitis and started on trimethoprim-sulfamethoxazole (Bactrim) DS 1 tab PO bid. The recommended action for the nurse practitioner is to:

    1. Instruct the client to continue Bactrim and see if any change occurs in the rash.

    2. Discontinue Bactrim.

    3. Take the client off Bactrim for 3 days and restart the medication.

    4. Decrease Bactrim to half dose.

23. When treating atopic dermatitis in children, all of the following instructions are applicable **except**:

    1. Eliminate one food that is thought to induce flares at a time.

    2. Avoid use of bubble bath.

    3. Avoid overheating.

    4. Encourage bathing two to three times a day.

24. An adolescent client complaining of hyperhidrosis should be counseled that: *excessive sweating*

    1. This is a normal occurrence.

    2. There are no therapies for this complaint.

    3. Bathing in a 20% alcohol solution of aluminum chloride hexahydrate (Drysol) on a nightly basis may be beneficial.

    4. A history and physical exam needs to be completed so that any medical etiologies can be ruled out.

25. What is the primary contributing factor to the development of diaper rash in an infant?

    1. Increased release of ammonia from the urine, increasing alkalinity, and irritation.

    2. Constant contact with wet diaper.

    3. Presence of *Candida albicans* on the skin.

    4. Urine and fecal enzymes together break down to form high alkaline levels.

26. An adolescent female presents with an irregular variegated nevus on her lower left back that has doubled in size in the past 3 months. The nurse practitioner should:

    1. Do a punch biopsy to confirm the diagnosis.

    2. Take a photograph of the lesion and recheck it in 1 month.

    3. Refer immediately to a dermatologist.

    4. Reassure the client that these are normal changes related to hormone variations.

27. An adolescent client presents with pain in his right chest wall for the past 48 hours. Upon examination, the nurse practitioner notices a vesicular eruption along the dermatome and identifies this as herpes zoster. The nurse practitioner informs the client:

    1. All symptoms will disappear in 3 days.

2. Oral medication can dramatically reduce the duration and intensity of symptoms.

3. He has chickenpox and can be contagious to his friends.

4. The eruptions will recur at regular intervals.

28. A young adolescent female presents to the nurse practitioner's office stating that she has a red rash over her trunk that itches and has been present for 2 weeks. She has tried over-the-counter lotions and creams, with no relief of symptoms. She states that it started as a small, round red patch on her chest and has since spread across her chest, back, arms, and legs. Physical exam reveals a generalized distribution of erythematous, scaly macular lesions that run parallel to each other, creating a "Christmas tree" pattern. The nurse practitioner should:

1. Do a thorough medication history, investigate any potential allergens, and send the client to an allergy specialist.

2. Prescribe triamcinolone acetonide 0.025% (Aristocort A) cream bid for 2 weeks.

3. Teach the adolescent client to expose herself to modest amounts of sunlight without burning, and use calamine lotion or oatmeal baths for symptom relief.

4. Refer the client to a dermatologist for a biopsy.

29. An adolescent male client presents to the nurse practitioner's office complaining of flu-like symptoms, a large red spot in the right groin, headaches, and generalized muscle pain. These symptoms have persisted for approximately 4–5 weeks. In taking the client's history, it would be most important to determine whether the client:

1. Was using new skin care products and detergents.

2. Was taking any new medications, vitamins or herbal therapies.

3. Has had a recent insect bite or potentially was exposed to insects such as ticks (i.e., camping trips, travel to heavily wooded areas).

4. Has been exposed to anyone who has tuberculosis.

30. A nurse practitioner is teaching the mother of a child how to use permethrin 1% creme rinse (Nix) for treatment of pediculosis capitis. What is the most important information the nurse practitioner should give to the mother?

1. Shampoo the child's hair daily for one week with permethrin 1% (Nix).

2. After hair is shampooed and towel-dried, apply permethrin 1% (Nix) creme rinse to scalp and hair, leaving on for 10 minutes before rinsing.

3. The shampoo should not be used again, as it is toxic and may absorb systemically and cause acute respiratory problems.

4. It is not necessary to treat other children in the family or launder bedding or clothing.

31. The nurse practitioner understands that most accidental scaldings in young children occur:

1. On the back of the body.

2. On the front of the body.

3. In a circular or glove pattern.

4. With no specific pattern.

32. An infant has pruritis due to eczema. The nurse practitioner teaches the mother the following regarding the infant's care:

1. Dress the infant in cotton shorts and short-sleeved shirts.

2. Dress the infant in wool blend long-sleeved jumpsuits.

3. Give the infant cornstarch or Aveeno baths.

4. Give the infant salt baths three times a day.

33. A new mother is concerned about the hemangioma on her infant's neck. What is the treatment choice for the majority of infants with hemangioma?

1. Cryosurgery.

2. Intralesional injection of steroids.

3. Observation.

4. Injection of a sclerosing agent.

34. The nurse practitioner is examining an infant with atopic dermatitis. The physical exam reveals:

    1. Dry, scaly rash with pruritis.

    2. Distribution of rash on face and extensor surfaces.

    3. Erythematous raised areas on flexor surfaces.

    4. Moist, crusting rash with no pruritis.

35. The practitioner is examining a 6-year-old child and identifies 8–10 patches of coffee-colored areas on the trunk. The areas are nontender, their borders are irregular, and most of the areas are >1.5 cm and are nonpalpable. What is the best recommendation to the parents of this child?

    1. The child should be further evaluated by a physician.

    2. These areas are normal pigmentation and will disappear.

    3. Suggest to the parents to consult a dermatologist for removal of lesions.

    4. Recommend emollients to keep skin moist and avoid sunlight on areas.

36. An infant is noted at his well-child visit to have a yellowish, greasy, scaly rash on his scalp, forehead, and ears. The most likely diagnosis would be:

    1. Seborrheic dermatitis.

    2. Atopic dermatitis.

    3. Erythema toxicum.

    4. Eczema.

37. A 1-month-old is being seen by the nurse practitioner for a diaper rash. Upon examination, the practitioner notes moderate erythema and poorly marginated, dry patches of skin that are localized to the buttocks. The deep folds are not affected. There are no satellite lesions. The most likely diagnosis would be:

    1. Infantile seborrheic dermatitis.

    2. Allergy to disposable diapers.

    3. Contact dermatitis.

    4. Candidal diaper rash.

38. The mother of a preschooler brings the child to see the nurse practitioner because of sores on his arms and legs. Upon examination, the nurse practitioner notes several honey-colored, crusted lesions with an erythematous base on the arms and legs. There is a history of exposure to mosquitoes. The rest of the physical examination is essentially negative. The most likely diagnosis would be:

    1. Scabies.

    2. Impetigo.

    3. Pityriasis rosea.

    4. Varicella.

39. A 6-month-old infant returns to the clinic to have his ears rechecked after a 10-day course of antibiotics for an ear infection. During the visit, the mother states that the child is now eating better and appears to be recovering, but he now has a bad diaper rash. The most likely cause of this rash is:

    1. Poor hygiene.

    2. Contact dermatitis.

    3. Seborrheic diaper dermatitis.

    4. *Candida albicans*.

40. A school-age child presents with erythematous papular lesions and scaly plaques in the antecubital and popliteal fossae and on the neck, wrists, and ankles. The mother states that the child has been scratching the areas, especially at night. History reveals that the child also has been treated for asthma. The nurse practitioner would make the diagnosis of:

    1. Scabies.

    2. Atopic dermatitis.

    3. Tinea corporis.

    4. Contact dermatitis.

# Childhood Diseases

41. Anticipatory guidance for the parents of a child with measles would include reporting the onset of which symptoms after the child begins recovery?

1. Fever, drowsiness, vomiting.

2. Skin desquamation.

3. Abdominal pain and diarrhea.

4. Worsening conjunctivitis.

42. A 6-year-old client with a rash on the face and Forschheimer spots on the soft palate will usually be diagnosed within 24 hours of the rash spread. The initial diagnosis may include:

    1. Rubella.

    2. Mononucleosis.

    3. Scarlet fever.

    4. All of the above.

43. Phone consultation with a mother reveals that her child has been on trimethoprim-sulfamethoxazole (Bactrim) for 3 days for a urinary tract infection. She has been treated with the drug previously with no problems. Currently, the child is experiencing blister-like sores in the skinfold areas (i.e., axilla and groin) as well as oral ulceration and a few sores in the genital area. Her temperature is 40°C and she is very weak. Differential diagnosis includes:

    1. Kawasaki's disease.

    2. Erythema multiforme (major).

    3. Viral exanthem.

    4. Early scalded skin syndrome.

44. A child's day care center director calls to confirm when the child can return to the center since the child had Fifth's disease (erythema infectiosum). The nurse practitioner's response is based on the knowledge that the period of communicability lasts until:

    1. The rash is gone.

    2. The rash appears.

    3. Upper respiratory symptoms are gone.

    4. The transient joint pain disappears.

45. Examination of an ill-appearing 6-year-old reveals vesicular and a few ulcerative oral lesions, an erythematous rash on the legs and buttocks with a maculopapular rash on the hands and feet, temperature of 38°C (100.4°F), and feelings of malaise. Differential diagnosis includes:

    1. Hand, foot, and mouth disease.

    2. Coxsackievirus, group B.

    3. ECHO virus 11.

    4. Varicella.

46. The clinical criteria for the diagnosis of Kawasaki's disease include:

    1. Unexplained low-grade fever, lasting several weeks.

    2. Prolonged, spiking fever from 101°F to 104°F that is unresponsive to antibiotics.

    3. Absence of rash or vesicular lesions.

    4. Decreased erythrocyte sedimentation rate (ESR) and hypochromic, microcytic anemia.

47. A child was diagnosed with varicella 3 days ago. The mother states that he started vomiting and has been "acting funny," staring off into space. Upon further questioning by the nurse practitioner, the vomiting was noted to be prolonged, effortless, and persistent. All of the following are to be considered in the differential diagnosis **except**:

    1. Encephalitis.

    2. Reye's syndrome.

    3. Drug poisoning.

    4. Anemia.

48. Which laboratory findings are associated with Reye's syndrome?

    1. Elevated aspartatate transaminase (AST) and alanine transaminase (ALT).

    2. Decreased serum ammonia.

    3. Hyperglycemia.

    4. Elevated bilirubin and shortened prothrombin time.

## Pharmacology

49. Which classification of drugs has the potential to aggravate psoriasis?

    1. β-Blockers.

    2. Thiazide diuretics.

    3. Vasodilators.

    4. Monoamine oxidase inhibitors.

50. In treatment of severe inflammatory acne for a female adolescent, the nurse practitioner understands that:

    1. Isotretinoin (Accutane) provides an effective first-line therapy.

    2. The benefits of treatment will be noted in 5–7 days.

    3. Counseling on stringent dietary changes is important.

    4. Systemic antibiotics are effective treatments.

51. A young mother brings her infant to the nurse practitioner with a complaint of difficulty with diaper rash. She reports the infant has had it for about a week. Upon exam, the diaper area appears beefy red with sharply marginated dermatitis. Satellite lesions are also noted. The family nurse recommends:

    1. Change from disposable diapers to cloth diapers with plastic pants.

    2. Application of nystatin (Mycostatin) after each diaper change.

    3. Apply wet soaks tid.

    4. Liberally apply oil after bathing.

52. An 8-year-old child presents to the clinic with a severe case of pediculosis. How would the nurse practitioner treat the problem in the eyebrows and eyelashes of the child? Teach the parent to:

    1. Apply petroleum jelly to lashes and brow 3–4 times a day.

    2. Apply neosporin ophthalmic ointment to the eyebrows and lashes.

    3. Apply a pediculicide to the lashes and eyebrows with a Q-tip.

4. Apply lindane ointment to the lashes and eyebrows.

53. When treating genital warts with topical podophyllin, it is important for the nurse practitioner to:

    1. Apply preparation directly to the wart and approximately 5 mm around base of wart.

    2. Cover with a dressing so the solution remains moist and caution client not to remove for 24 hours.

    3. Instruct client to wash off medication in 4–6 hours.

    4. Treat with liquid nitrogen before applying podophyllin.

54. When using lidocaine with epinephrine 1–2% as a local anesthetic in the repair of an injury, it is essential to keep in mind that the maximum allowable dose is:

    1. 7 mg/kg.

    2. 2 mg/kg.

    3. 10 mg/kg.

    4. 5 mg/kg.

55. On a return visit to the clinic, a child who is receiving sulfonamide therapy exhibits the following symptoms: generalized rash, mucous membrane lesions, sloughing of the skin of the palms and feet, high fever, and generalized malaise. These findings would alert the nurse practitioner to consider:

    1. Hepatitis B.

    2. Stevens-Johnson syndrome.

    3. HIV infection/acquired immunodeficiency syndrome.

    4. *Pneumocystis carinii* pneumonia.

56. The nurse practitioner is examining lesions on a child's face around his nose and mouth. The mother states the lesions began several days ago and seem to be getting worse. The lesions are vesicular, edematous, red, and tender. Some have yellow crusts and an erythematous base. The treatment for this child is:

1. Mupirocin ointment (Bactroban) qid × 10 days.

2. Gently soaking the lesions with antibacterial soap and removing the crust.

3. Dicloxacillin (Dynapen) at 15 mg/kg/day divided into four doses × 10 days.

4. Diphenhydramine HCl (Benadryl) 5 mg PO q6h to decrease itching and spreading.

57. The mother a 1-year-old child brings the child to the clinic for problems with a "rash." She states the child has not been feeling well since the rash started 2 days ago. The nurse practitioner observes numerous macules and vesicles in clusters over the child's trunk and mucous membranes; some are clear and some are crusting. The child is irritable but does not have a fever. The diagnosis and treatment for this child include:

1. Varicella; immunize with varicella zoster vaccine to decrease symptoms and begin acyclovir (Zovirax) therapy to decrease incidence of severe complications.

2. Impetigo; treat with antibiotics for 10 days and return to clinic in 2 weeks.

3. Contact dermatitis; thoroughly review with mother any changes in care, diphenhydramine HCl (Benadryl) spray over the rash, cut child's fingernails to decrease scratching.

4. Varicella; treat with hydroxyzine (Atarax) 2 mg/kg/day in three divided doses for itching, daily baths with baking soda to relieve itching and prevent superinfection.

58. A six-month-old is brought to the clinic for a rash on the face and diaper area that consists of linear erythematous burrows. An older sibling has a similar rash on his wrists and between his fingers. An appropriate intervention would be:

1. Neosporin ointment.

2. Mycitracin ointment.

3. Acitretin (Soriatane).

4. Permethrin 5% cream (Elimite).

59. A mother brings her school-age child to the nurse practitioner's office. She states that the child developed a blistering rash on his face 2 days ago that has since spread to his hands and forearms. Examination reveals the presence of multiple, small vesicular lesions across the child's face, arms, and hands. Some of the lesions are covered with a honey-colored crust. The nurse practitioner diagnoses impetigo and:

1. Recommends frequent scrubbing of the lesions with a stiff-bristled brush.

2. Recommends keeping the child isolated for 7 days and discarding clothing the child has been wearing since the lesions appeared.

3. Prescribes dicloxacillin (Dynapen) suspension, 25 mg/kg/day, divided into four doses × 10 days, and recommends gentle washing of the lesions to remove any loose crusts, and washing the child's clothing and linen separately in hot water.

4. Refers the child to a dermatologist and counsels the mother that she needs to practice better personal hygiene.

60. An adolescent female presents to the nurse practitioner's office with a prolonged history of facial acne. She has been seen by several dermatologists and has been treated over the past 3 years with multiple therapies, including topical antibiotics, drying agents, intralesional injections of corticosteroids, and multiple systemic antibiotics, without success. After consulting with the collaborating physician, the nurse practitioner prescribes isotretinoin (Accutane). Teaching/counseling related to the use of this medication includes:

1. No dietary/alcohol restrictions are necessary.

2. Exposure to sunlight without burning can be helpful in hastening the healing process.

3. Eliminate all fat from the client's diet.

4. Emphasize the importance of using effective contraception if the client is sexually active, due to the teratogenicity of the drug.

61. Indications for the use of oral acyclovir within 24 hours of rash eruption in children with chickenpox are:

    1. Child over the age of 6.

    2. Chronic neurologic disorders.

    3. Use of aerosolized corticosteroids.

    4. Concomitant otitis media.

62. The medication of choice in treating Kawasaki's disease is:

    1. Prednisone during the acute phase.

    2. Intravenous gamma globulin (IVGG).

    3. Acetaminophen (Tylenol).

    4. Low-dose aspirin during the acute phase.

# 8  Answers & Rationales

## Physical Examination & Diagnostic Tests

1. **(4)** Annular skin lesions may be arranged in a circular manner or in an arciform (arc) pattern (i.e., tinea corporis). Multiple groups of vesicles erupting unilaterally following the course of cutaneous nerves is herpetiform or zosteriform (i.e., herpes zoster). Linear lesions are arranged in a line (i.e., allergic contact dermatitis to poison ivy). Confluent lesions become merged together and are not discrete (i.e., scarlet fever rash).

2. **(1)** The place to inspect is in that portion of the sclera that is observed when the eye is open. If jaundice is suspected, the posterior portion of the hard palate should be examined for a yellowish cast. Pallor and cyanosis can be noted in the nail beds, palms, and soles.

3. **(1)** Fungal lesions will be visualized as a green–yellow fluorescence when viewed with the Wood's light in a dim room.

4. **(1)** A macule is less than 1 cm in diameter, nonpalpable, and brown, red, purple, or tan (freckles, flat moles, rubella). A papule is elevated and palpable (warts, pigmented nevi). A nodule is 1–2 cm diameter, elevated, and deeper (lipoma). A wheal is elevated and irregular and has a variable diameter (insect bites, urticaria).

5. **(2)** Lichenification occurs with chronic irritation, often of an exposed extremity (chronic dermatitis). Crusts are dried exudate; scales are heaps of keratinized cells from exfoliation (psoriasis); and loss of epidermis is excoriation, as seen in an abrasion.

6. **(3)** The angle of the nail beds should form a diamond when the nail beds are approximated. Transverse ridges and grooves may occur from trauma. Placing the palms together provides no assessment data, and diffuse discoloration may be from a fungal infection or an injury.

7. **(3)** Bulla is the correct terminology. A papule is solid, a vesicle is <1 cm in diameter, and a pustule contains a purulent exudate.

8. **(4)** The appearance of a new mole with high-risk features, including irregular border, color changes, and changes in sensation (i.e., pruritis), would necessitate immediate biopsy to rule out melanoma and/or referral to a dermatologist. Uniform moles, those that are symmetrical and have smooth borders, and those that are not showing signs of change are those that can be followed with annual skin assessments. Seborrheic keratosis is a benign skin growth that usually presents on sun-exposed areas and appears waxy or "stuck on," requiring no treatment.

9. **(2)** Under microscope exam, fungal scrapings in KOH solution will appear as thread-like hyphae crossing cell walls. The other solutions are not indicated for use to identify dermatophytes.

10. **(3)** It is important to remember to apply controls when skin testing the immunocompromised client. Ask clients what diseases they believe they have immunity to, such as measles. Apply the "known" allergen and the skin test to be tested. If the client is unable to mount an immune response at all, the known allergen will not react. By not applying the controls, the nurse practitioner may assume a skin test is negative when in fact the client's immune system is unable to respond.

11. **(4)** This best describes Mongolian spots, which are characteristic in newborns of African, Asian, or Latin descent. When closely evaluated, these spots do not have the appearance of ecchymoses that occur with trauma. Telangiectatic nevi are commonly known as "stork bites" and are deep pink lesions most often found on back of the neck. Cutis marmorata is the transient mottling that occurs when an infant is cold.

# Skin Disorders

12. **(3)** Intense itching is characteristic of pediculosis pubis, scabies, and atopic dermatitis. Impetigo starts out as a tender erythematous papule and progresses through a vesicular to a honey-crusted stage with no itching.

13. **(2)** Herpes zoster typically presents with history of tenderness followed by eruptions and vesicles that follow a dermatome on one side of the body. This is very painful. Other symptoms may include fever, headaches, and malaise.

14. **(2)** Approximately 10–30% of people with psoriasis develop an accompanying form of arthritis called psoriatic arthritis. The other options are dermatologic conditions but are not directly associated with arthritis.

15. **(3)** Stress can aggravate psoriasis. Sunlight helps psoriasis, so it is usually better in the summer. It is not contagious and only about 30% of clients with psoriasis itch.

16. **(1)** The location and appearance of the lesions is typical of scabies—short, irregular runs approximately 2–3 mm long and the width of a hair.

17. **(4)** Laboratory studies are not likely to be helpful in evaluation of urticaria. Identification of causes is usually based on history and physical findings. The other statements are true of urticaria.

18. **(3)** Although any one of these skin conditions can affect the skin particularly of an HIV-positive client, the description relates most closely to Kaposi's sarcoma and warrants a biopsy.

19. **(2)** Despite the name dyshidrotic eczematous dermatitis (bullous form called pompholyx), there is no evidence of sweating. Most clients have an atopic history, and emotional stress is often a precipitating factor to the appearance of the vesicles. Nummular (discoid) eczema is a chronic, pruritic, inflammatory dermatitis that occurs in the form of coin-shaped plaques composed of grouped small papules and vesicles on an erythematous base. Option #1 describes rosacea. Option #3 describes psoriasis. Option #4 describes a verruca or common wart.

20. **(4)** Delay wound closure until determination of no infection in approximately 24–48 hours. Mouth flora of humans is abundant and, with a bite, there is the possibility for heavy bacterial inoculum and potential severe infection. Tetanus toxoid is indicated since there has been no booster in the last 5 years.

21. **(2)** Onychomycosis is the correct term. Hippocratic nails are clubbed nails and fingers associated with chronic heart and lung disorders; koilonychia is a concavity of the nail plate often associated with iron deficiency anemia; and anonychia is a total congenital absence of the nail.

22. **(2)** In cases of suspected drug reactions, it is recommended the drug be eliminated and documented in the client's record so it is not reintroduced.

23. **(4)** Excessive bathing dries the skin, which irritates the atopic dermatitis. Food allergies, along with any other causative triggers, should be identified and avoided. Bubble bath can irritate skin, as can sweating.

24. **(4)** Excessive sweating can be normal, but the client needs to have a history and physical to rule out any underlying causes. There are therapies that can be offered. The Drysol is only for use on feet and axillae. Full bathing is not recommended with this solution.

25. **(4)** All factors listed do contribute, however the combination of urine and stool causes excessive alkalinity and makes it more irritating than the urine alone.

26. **(3)** Refer immediately to a dermatologist since these are highly suspicious findings of a melanoma. Biopsy should never be done on a melanoma, and any delay in time could be detrimental to the outcome.

27. **(2)** Oral acyclovir is very effective in reducing intensity and duration of symptoms if started early in the course of the disease. Herpes zoster does not usually recur at regular intervals, but it frequently lasts for several weeks.

28. **(3)** This client presents with a classic case of pityriasis rosea, a benign, self-limiting skin eruption of unknown etiology. Although a medication/allergen history would be warranted, referral to an allergy specialist or dermatologist would not be necessary. Triamcinolone would not be indicated as the treatment is mainly symptomatic. Sunlight in moderate amounts has been shown to hasten healing in some cases.

29. **(3)** The signs and symptoms presented are classic for Lyme disease, which is transmitted by ticks. Therefore, it would be important to inquire about potential exposure to ticks in the time period prior to the development of signs and symptoms. Exposure to new skin care products would be important if the practitioner suspected an allergic reaction, which is not consistent with the signs and symptoms presented. While a thorough medication history should always be done, it is most likely not going to reveal the cause of the signs and

symptoms in this case. Tuberculosis does not present in this manner.

30. **(2)** This is the correct procedure for the shampoo, e.g., after hair is shampooed and towel-dried, apply permethrin 1% (Nix) creme rinse to scalp and hair, leaving on for 10 minutes before rinsing. After the rinse, remove nits with a nit comb. Repeat shampoo treatment after 7 days, if living lice still observed. Clothing and bedding should be washed or drycleaned. Family members should also be treated.

31. **(2)** Accidental scalding is usually splash-related and occurs on the front of the body. The nurse practitioner should be suspicious of any burns on the back of the body or any well-defined, uniform burn areas on the buttocks or extremities, as they may indicate physical abuse. Immersion burns on the buttocks may be seen as punishment for toileting or wetting "accidents."

32. **(3)** The cornstarch or Aveeno baths will temporarily help relieve the itching. The shorts and short-sleeved shirt would expose too much skin, which would be scratched by the infant. Wool irritates the skin. Salt would also be an irritant.

33. **(3)** The most common treatment is to observe, as the majority of hemangiomas resolve within time, usually beginning around 18 months of age. The other treatments may be performed, especially for those that are proliferating at a fast rate.

34. **(2)** Infantile atopic dermatitis, as contrasted with atopic dermatitis in older children and adolescents, is a moist, oozing, crusting rash with pruritis found mainly on the extensor surfaces of the body and the face. It usually begins around 2 months of age, and often there is a family history of atopy.

35. **(1)** In prepubertal children, café au lait spots that are greater than 1 cm and are present in more than five areas are of concern as they may be associated with neurofibromatosis. The child should be referred to a pediatrician for further evaluation.

36. **(1)** Seborrheic dermatitis is usually salmon colored and has a yellowish, greasy appearance. It occurs in infants <6 months of age. It does not itch. The distribution is mainly to the face, postauricular scalp, axillae, and groin. Atopic dermatitis and eczema are pink or red if inflamed and have a whiter, nongreasy appearance. They may begin at 2–12 months and continue through childhood, and are associated with a family history of allergy. The distribution is to the cheeks, trunk, and extensors of the extremities. Itching may be severe. Erythema toxicum consists of yellow or white papules on the face. It occurs in 30–50% of term infants and disappears in 2 weeks.

37. **(3)** Given the distribution of the rash, the most likely cause is a contact dermatitis such as that caused by the use of baby wipes. Allergy to disposable diapers would involve the entire diaper area. Seborrheic dermatitis presents as large, confluent, sharply marginated, bright plaques on the anterior surface of the groin. Candidal rashes are bright red with satellite lesions that involve the deep folds and may spread to the entire diaper area.

38. **(2)** Impetigo presents with honey-colored, crusted lesions with an erythematous base. Staphylococci and group A streptococci are important pathogens in this disease. Scabies presents with linear burrows about the wrists, ankles, finger webs, areolae, anterior axillary folds, genitals, or face (in infants). Pityriasis rosea presents as erythematous papules that coalesce to form oval plaques preceded by a large oval plaque with central clearing and a scaly border (the herald patch). Varicella presents as crops of red macules that rapidly become tiny vesicles with surrounding erythema that form pustules. The pustules become crusted and then scab over. The rash appears predominantly on the trunk and face.

39. **(4)** After a course of antibiotics, the normal flora are destroyed, making the child a prime target for *Candida albicans*. The classic signs of a yeast infection include a beefy red, sharply marginated, maculopapular rash with satellite lesions. Poor hygiene or a contact dermatitis would present as erythema and thickening of the skin in the perianal area. Seborrheic dermatitis consists of an erythematous, scaly dermatitis accompanied by overproduction of sebum occurring in areas rich in sebaceous glands (i.e., the face, scalp, and perineum).

40. **(2)** Atopic dermatitis commonly presents in the flexural areas of children. The lesions are characteristically erythematous and papular, with scales and pruritis commonly noted. A personal or family history of atopy is noted in about 70% of clients with atopic dermatitis. Scabies lesions appear as gray or skin-colored ridges, vesicles, and papules. Tinea corporis lesions are generally distributed over the entire body and face and have an area of clearing in the center of the lesion. Contact dermatitis usually produces lesions in the shape of the object causing the reaction, and are usually vesicular in nature.

# Childhood Diseases

41. **(1)** Fever, drowsiness, vomiting, headache, convulsions, and possible coma are signs of neurologic complications that present as the child appears to recover.

42. **(4)** Rubella may be difficult to diagnose, and the rash is often confused with infectious mononucleosis and scarlet fever.

43. **(2)** Kawasaki's disease presents with a more diffuse erythematous rash. Viral exanthems are centrally located and not blister-like. Scalded skin syndrome, staphylococcal in origin, causes the skin to peel off and be very red. Erythema multiform is a major side effect of sulfa drug use that presents with a sudden onset of high fever, weakness, blisters, bullae, and ulcerations of the mucous membranes.

44. **(2)** The incubation period for erythema infectiosum is 4–14 days, with communicability until the rash appears.

45. **(1)** The symptoms are indicative of coxsackievirus 5 or 16, group A, which is called hand, foot, and mouth disease.

Varicella lesions begin on the trunk with classic "teardrop vesicles."

46. **(2)** Fever is the only universal sign of Kawasaki's disease (i.e., prolonged, spiking fever from 101°F to 104°F that is unresponsive to antibiotics). Other symptoms include nonexudative conjuctivitis; inflammation of the oral mucosa (strawberry tongue and dry, erythematous, cracked lips); nonvesicular, diffuse rash involving trunk and extremities; cervical lymphadenopathy (usually unilateral in the anterior cervical chain); edema and erythema of the palms and soles followed later by desquamation starting on the fingertips; and deep, linear, transverse nail grooves (Beau's lines) in the convalescent stage. Cardiovascular dysfunction may develop (e.g., myocarditis, coronary aneurysm). Laboratory findings include increased ESR and white blood cell count; normocytic, normochromic anemia; and elevated platelet count.

47. **(4)** Any disorder that can impair neurologic functioning and alter hepatic function can be considered in the differential diagnosis of Reye's syndrome. In addition, drug overdose, head trauma, toxic ingestion of chemicals, poisoning, diabetic coma, or renal failure have symptoms similar to Reye's syndrome.

48. **(1)** Elevated AST (SGOT) and ALT (SGPT) at least three times normal, hypoglycemia, and increased serum ammonia, blood urea nitrogen, and creatinine are found in Reye's syndrome. The bilirubin is usually normal or slightly elevated and the prothrombin time is lengthened.

## Pharmacology

49. **(1)** β-Blockers can exacerbate psoriasis. They are believed to decrease cyclic-AMP–dependent protein kinase (an inhibitor of cell proliferation). There is no known effect with the other stated classifications.

50. **(4)** Systemic antibiotics (such as tetracycline) offer the most effective treatment in inflammatory acne. Accutane is also very effective but, because of serious teratogenic side effects, it is not first-line treatment. Improvement in acne will not be noted for 4–8 weeks, and dietary changes have not been demonstrated to have any beneficial effect.

51. **(2)** Appearance is indicative of *Candida albicans*, which is best treated with nystatin. The other choices would aggravate the diaper rash due to promotion of overhydration.

52. **(1)** The petroleum jelly is thought to smother the lice. Pediculicide should not be applied to the face close to the eyes, and neosporin ointment will not kill the lice.

53. **(3)** Clients need to be instructed to wash off podophyllin. It is to be applied sparingly, only to the wart while avoiding normal skin, and allowed to dry thoroughly before the client dresses. There is no rationale to treat with both liquid nitrogen and podophyllin.

54. **(1)** The correct answer is 7 mg/kg for lidocaine with epinephrine for children and 5 mg/kg for lidocaine without epinephrine. Although local anesthetics are commonly used, the maximum allowable doses are rarely emphasized, and overdose can result in anaphylactic shock.

55. **(2)** Stevens-Johnson syndrome is a severe form of erythema multiforme that can be fatal. The clinical picture of this syndrome is mucous membrane lesions, conjunctival and corneal lesions, fever, malaise, arthralgia, and sloughing of the skin of the hands and feet. The distinguishing characteristics that differentiate this condition are the eruption of vesicles and ulcerations of the mucosa and the sloughing skin.

56. **(3)** The child's lesions are characteristic of impetigo and should be treated with an antibiotic. If they are present on the child's face, dicloxacillin is the drug of choice. The ointment, the soaking, and the Benadryl will not stop the spread of the infection, which could lead to poststreptococcal glomerulonephritis.

57. **(4)** Varicella (chickenpox) should be treated symptomatically unless the child is at high risk secondary to other medical problems. Acyclovir is not recommended for routine treatment of uncomplicated varicella. Impetigo commonly occurs on the face and neck and usually does not have diffuse lesions over the trunk. Contact dermatitis is characterized by erythema and scaling and may have weeping vesicles; area of distribution of rash offers clues to diagnosis.

58. **(4)** Permethrin 5% cream (Elimite) is used in infants; however, it is not recommended in those under 2 months of age. Neosporin could be used to treat secondary infections but would do nothing to eradicate the scabies. Mycitracin is also not effective for the treatment of scabies. Acitretin (Soriatane) is used for the treatment of psoriasis.

59. **(3)** Impetigo is communicable until the client has been on antibiotic therapy for 48 hours. Washing clothing and linens separately with hot water is recommended, along with surveillance of close contacts for the appearance of lesions. Isolation is not necessary, except to keep the child home from school until 48 hours of antibiotic therapy have been completed. Dicloxacillin is considered to be the drug of choice. Gentle washing is recommended to keep the lesions clean and to prevent scarring (potentially caused by vigorous scrubbing).

60. **(4)** Isotretinoin is extremely teratogenic; therefore, a sexual assessment, along with a pregnancy test in women with child-bearing capacity and contraceptive counseling, should be done for all clients. The combination of alcohol and isotretinoin can cause a disulfiram-like reaction; therefore, the use of alcohol should be avoided. Isotretinoin can cause photosensitivity, so the nurse practitioner should counsel the client to avoid sunlight, wear protective clothing and sunglasses, and apply sunscreen to all sun-exposed areas without acne. No conclusive relationship between diet and acne has been established.

61. **(3)** The indications for use of oral acyclovir in chickenpox are that the child is over age 12, has a chronic pulmonary disorder, is on chronic salicylate therapy, or is receiving an intermittent or short courses of aerosolized corticosteroids.

62. **(2)** Current medication therapy includes the use of high-dose aspirin (80–100 mg/kg/day qid) until the child is afebrile; then the dose is reduced to 3–5 mg/kg/day in a single dose. If varicella or influenza develop, then the aspirin therapy is discontinued to prevent development of Reye's syndrome. IVGG is administered during the acute phase of the disease. Steroid use is contraindicated as steroids have not been shown to prevent the development of coronary aneurysms.

# Endocrine

## Physical Examination & Diagnostic Tests

1. What is the correct procedure for palpation of a child's thyroid gland?

   1. Stand behind the child, hyperextend the head, and palpate both sides simultaneously.

   2. Have the child lower his chin and lean his head slightly toward the side being evaluated.

   3. Hyperextend the head and have the child lean away from the side being evaluated.

   4. Have the child lead away from the side being examined and take a swallow of water.

2. When a child sips water and swallows, the thyroid gland:

   1. Moves downward and slightly posterior and feels smooth on palpation.

   2. Elongates and enlarges during the swallow and immediately returns to a resting position at the end of palpation.

   3. Moves slightly out during the sipping and backward during the swallowing.

   4. Moves upward during the swallow and feels symmetrical and smooth to palpation.

3. When doing a physical examination on a child with hyperthyroidism, a common neurologic finding is:

   1. Memory, attention, and problem-solving deficits.

   2. Diminished deep tendon reflexes.

   3. Severe cognitive impairment.

   4. Delusions and psychosis.

4. Which finding would alert the nurse practitioner that a client might be experiencing a problem with the endocrine system?

   1. Coagulation abnormalities and fatigue.

   2. Growth abnormalities and glucose intolerance.

   3. Hypoxia and jaundice.

   4. Steatorrhea and abdominal distention.

5. The nurse practitioner notes a solitary thyroid nodule on a client during a routine physical examination. The preferred diagnostic test of choice is:

   1. Thyroid scan and antibody level.
   2. Thyroid-stimulating hormone (TSH) and ultrasound.
   3. X-ray of the thyroid.
   4. Fine-needle aspiration biopsy.

6. In evaluating the laboratory values taken from a client with Graves' disease, one should expect:

   1. TSH levels to be increased.
   2. TSH levels to be decreased.
   3. TSH levels to be within normal limits.
   4. Thyroxine ($T_4$) levels to be decreased.

## Disorders

7. The etiology of type I diabetes can be best described as:

   1. An autosomal dominant genetic disorder.
   2. Autoimmune destruction of the β cells.
   3. Overnutrition and resulting obesity as the major risk factor.
   4. Prevented by exercise, which increases the concentration of insulin receptors.

8. Hirsutism presenting in a young female with normal menstruation and normal plasma androgens is most likely:

   1. An ovarian tumor.
   2. Cushing's syndrome.
   3. Idiopathic.
   4. Polycystic ovary disease.

9. Pathophysiologic reasons for decreased testosterone level develop in the:

   1. Hypothalamus, posterior pituitary.
   2. Anterior pituitary, adrenals, testes.
   3. Testes, adrenals, posterior pituitary.
   4. Hypothalamus, anterior pituitary, testes.

10. The most common cause of poor control of type I diabetics during the adolescent period is:

    1. Emotional disturbance.
    2. Noncompliance with dietary restrictions.
    3. Poor adherence to blood testing and insulin injections.
    4. All of the above.

11. A goal in the management of a 7-year-old child with diabetes would be to maintain the blood sugar in what range?

    1. 100–200 mg/dl.
    2. 80–180 mg/dl.
    3. 70–150 mg/dl.
    4. 80–120 mg/dl.

12. A mother presents her school-age child to the nurse practitioner and expresses her concern that her son is the shortest child in his class and asks if something is the matter with him. Initial differentiation of cause of the child's short stature by the nurse practitioner would include:

    1. History and physical exam, including Tanner stage with possible skeletal maturation assessed by radiography, if indicated.
    2. History, physical exam, and trial treatment with growth hormone.
    3. Immediate referral to an endocrinologist.
    4. Physical exam and complete blood count, thyroid function panel, urinalysis, karotyping, chemistry profile, and insulin sensitivity tests.

13. Which of the following findings would the nurse practitioner expect to find in a child with pubertal gynecomastia?

    1. Tanner stage II with testes ≤4 cm in length.

2. Breasts and nipples nontender and equal in size.

3. Breast tissue enlargement mainly glandular, movable, and nonadherent to skin or underlying tissue.

4. Lymphadenopathy, goiter, asymmetrical testes, and repaired hypospadias.

14. Which of the following is true regarding hyperthyroidism in children?

1. Boys have a higher incidence of Graves' disease.

2. Autoimmune response is most often triggered by the body's reaction to a bacterial or viral infection.

3. There is decreased production and secretion of thyroid hormone and presence of goiter.

4. It is a common, endemic congenital disorder caused by iodine deficiency.

15. The nurse practitioner notes the following on physical examination of a 14-year-old adolescent who complains of amenorrhea: blood pressure 138/90, pulse 98, broad chest with widely spaced nipples, Tanner stage I, webbing of neck, low hairline, and prominent, anomalous ears. The nurse practitioner suspects:

1. Klinefelter's syndrome.

2. Marfan's syndrome.

3. Fragile X syndrome.

4. Turner's syndrome.

16. The nurse practitioner understands that growth retardation that appears after age 12 in boys is usually due to:

1. Chromosomal abnormalities.

2. Hyperthyroidism.

3. Hyperpituitarism.

4. Hypogonadism.

17. Which of the following conditions is associated with growth failure?

1. Fanconi's syndrome.

2. Tourette's syndrome.

3. Klinefelter's syndrome.

4. Angelman's syndrome.

18. Assessment of diabetic ketoacidosis in a child is often confusing because of the high frequency of which symptom?

1. Joint pain.

2. Cheyne-Stokes breathing.

3. Diaphoresis.

4. Abdominal pain.

19. An adolescent male presenting with recent-onset nocturia, polydipsia, polyphagia, weight loss, and blurred vision is most likely to be experiencing the symptoms of:

1. Insulin-dependent diabetes mellitus (IDDM).

2. Non–insulin-dependent diabetes mellitus (NIDM).

3. Urinary tract infection (UTI).

4. Mononucleosis.

20. In which of the following groups of clients is tight glycemic control contraindicated?

1. Adolescent males.

2. Adolescent females.

3. Children 9–12 years.

4. Infants under 2.

21. An infant with an abnormally pitched cry may demonstrate a genetic disorder or other problems such as:

1. Hypothyroidism.

2. Hypertelorism.

3. Cleft palate.

4. Pyloric stenosis.

# Pharmacology

22. An infant with congenital hypothyroidism is being given levothyroxine (Synthroid). The nurse practitioner would instruct the parents to:

    1. Watch for constipation and slow pulse as signs of toxicity.

    2. Reduce the medication as symptoms decrease.

    3. Give the medication as a single dose in the early morning.

    4. Expect weight loss until the child adjusts to the dose.

23. A 6-year-old child with hypothyroidism diagnosed shortly after birth is seen by the nurse practitioner for a routine physical exam. His temperature is 96.8°F (36°C) and his pulse is 68. The mother states that she has noticed that the child has been constipated and seems to be more tired than usual. Based on the history of this child, the nurse practitioner should suspect:

    1. The child has been taking too much of his levothyroxine (Synthroid) and is exhibiting symptoms of toxicity.

    2. The child needs to add more fluids to his diet to correct his constipation.

    3. The child needs to have his dose of levothyroxine (Synthroid) increased because he is exhibiting signs of hypothyroidism.

    4. The child has "outgrown" his hypothyroidism and no longer needs levothyroxine (Synthroid).

24. A 6-year-old has been discharged home on desmopressin acetate (DDAVP) for diabetes insipidus after a pituitary tumor removal. Upon examination, it is noted that the child is lethargic but has 4+ deep tendon reflexes. The nurse practitioner suspects:

    1. Noncompliance with therapy.

    2. Water intoxication.

    3. Increased vasopressor effect.

    4. Interaction with over-the-counter cough medicine products.

25. When monitoring an adolescent's insulin therapy regimen, the nurse practitioner is aware that the NPH to Regular insulin proportions are:

    1. 2:1 in the AM and 1:1 in the PM.

    2. 1:1 in the AM and 1:2 in the PM.

    3. 1:2 in the AM and 2:1 in the PM.

    4. 1:1 in the AM and PM.

26. The nurse practitioner understands that lispro insulin (Humalog):

    1. Can be injected just prior to eating.

    2. Is less costly than regular insulin.

    3. Increases the likelihood of late postprandial hypoglycemia due to its length of action.

    4. Has a long-term safety profile and does not cause any teratogenic effects.

27. Which statement is correct concerning anabolic–androgenic steroid use in adolescents?

    1. Promotes physical growth and enhances sexual activity.

    2. Produces premature epiphyseal closure.

    3. Causes an increase in breast development in females.

    4. Increases testicular size.

28. Which is the medical treatment of choice of hyperinsulinism in infants?

    1. Glucagon 20–30 µg/kg.

    2. Regular insulin 10 units IV.

    3. Glucose IV at 12–14 mg/kg/min.

    4. Methylprednisolone (Medrol) 0.6 mg/kg/day.

29. The nurse practitioner understands that growth hormone (somatropin or Genotropin) is administered:

    1. By subcutaneous injection into the thigh, buttocks, or abdomen.

    2. By intravenous monthly injections.

    3. Only after the child's epiphyses are closed or fused.

4. By oral suspension in 5 mg/mL preparation.

30. A child with Grave's disease is being treated with methimazole (Tapazole). What is a serious potential side effect?

1. Purpuric, papular rash.

2. Alopecia.

3. Agranulocytosis. (leukopenia)

4. Joint pain.

Treat hyperthyroidism ( ↓ TSH, ↑T3/T4, grave's ds)
c̄ Tapazole/ PTU

# 9   Answers & Rationales

## Physical Examination & Diagnostic Tests

1. **(2)** When examining the thyroid, it is important to have the child relax the sternocleidomastoid muscles. This can be done by having the client lean toward the side being evaluated.

2. **(4)** The thyroid gland is fixed to the trachea and thus ascends during swallowing. This assists the nurse practitioner to distinguish thyroid structures from other neck masses. The gland's size, degree of enlargement, consistency, surface characteristics, and presence of nodules or bruits are noted during the examination.

3. **(1)** The high level of thyroid hormone affects the nervous system, causing sympathomimetic symptoms such as brisk deep tendon reflexes; fine, rapid tremor of the hands; restlessness; irritability; insomnia; dreams; nightmares; and rarely severe cognitive impairment and psychosis.

4. **(2)** Growth abnormalities are associated with anterior pituitary dysfunction and glucose intolerance with diabetes related to pancreas dysfunction. Coagulation abnormalities and fatigue would be associated with hematologic dysfunction. Hypoxia would be associated with oxygenation problems and jaundice with liver or biliary problems. Steatorrhea is associated with malabsorption syndrome and cystic fibrosis.

5. **(4)** Although the primary care provider may obtain TSH and antibody levels, the preferred diagnostic tool for the endocrinologist is the fine-needle aspiration biopsy. Scans, sonography, and x-ray tests can be used in initial screening; they do not assist in the determination of whether the nodule is malignant or not. The aspirate is sent for cytology and interpretation.

6. **(2)** TSH levels should be decreased in a client with Graves' disease because thyroid-stimulating immunoglobulins bind to TSH receptors, which increases $T_4$ synthesis and release, subsequently suppressing TSH levels.

## Disorders

7. **(2)** Type I diabetes is caused by destruction of the $\beta$ cells mediated through the immune system. The other three choices refer to type II diabetes.

8. **(3)** Because of the normal menstrual periods and androgen plasma level, this would be considered idiopathic. Diseases related to the ovaries would cause changes in the menstrual cycle, and with Cushing's syndrome there would be adrenal androgen overproduction.

9. **(4)** Testosterone production is regulated by the hypothalamic–pituitary–testicular (HPT) axis. Thus abnormalities in any one of these areas can affect the production of testosterone.

10. **(4)** All of these contribute significantly to difficulty in controlling diabetes in the teen years. Hormonal changes and the desire to become independent increase emotional conflicts. Teens have a great desire to be like their peers and do not want to be regimented in following a specific diet and adhering to a treatment plan.

11. **(2)** Children between 5 and 12 years, 80–180 mg/dl; children <5, 100–200 mg/dl; and children 13 years and older, 70–150 mg/dl. Normal levels are 80–120 mg/dl.

12. **(1)** This is the best choice for the initial exam since the history may reveal normal variation in pattern of growth related to race, heredity, size of other family members, and psychosocial status. Skeletal maturation ("bone age") can be assessed through radiography, if child is less than or equal to the fifth growth percentile. The other choices are inappropriate without history and physical exam, and growth hormone would not be administered without lab evaluation.

13. **(3)** Pubertal (physiologic) gynecomastia is a visible or palpable glandular enlargement of the male breast that can occur in healthy adolescents. Typically, the breasts are unequal in size, and may be tender; the nipples are often irritated secondary to rubbing against clothing; and Tanner stages II to IV of pubertal development are noted. The symptoms in Option #4 are associated with pathologic gynecomastia.

14. **(2)** Hyperthyroidism in children most commonly affects girls and is an autoimmune disorder (Graves' disease) in which the body produces antibodies that stimulate TSH receptors, causing an overproduction of thyroid hormones and goiter. Hypothyroidism is associated with iodine deficiency.

15. **(4)** These findings are consistent with Turner's syndrome—short stature, gonadal dysgenesis, lymphedema (usually appearing in infancy), left-sided heart or aortic abnormalities, primary amenorrhea, and delayed onset of puberty. Fragile X syndrome is an inherited condition usually affecting males and characterized by long narrow face and prominent ears, mild to profound mental retardation, hyperactivity and poor attention span, and autistic-type behavior. Marfan's syndrome is a connective tissue disorder in the adolescent who is tall and thin, and is characterized by long limbs, narrow hands, long slender fingers, and nearsightedness. Klinefelter's syndrome is characterized by small testes, sterility, gynecomastia, and long legs.

16. **(4)** Hypogonadism characterized by delayed sexual development, sexual infantilism, and small testes is most often the contributing factor to growth retardation after age 10 years for girls and 12 years for boys. Other causes of decelerated growth or short stature include hypothyroidism, diabetes, and hypopituitarism. Chromosomal abnormalities would be noted at an earlier age.

17. **(1)** Fanconi's syndrome is most often a hereditary problem caused by an inborn error of metabolism, such as galactosemia or Wilson's disease, and usually presents as growth failure in children. Tourette's syndrome is a disorder characterized by multiple vocal or motor tics. Angelman's syndrome is a disorder characterized by mental retardation, seizures, wide-based ataxic gait, and a pleasant, happy disposition with limited vocabulary or absent speech. Klinefelter's syndrome is characterized by small testes, sterility, gynecomastia, and long legs.

18. **(4)** Abdominal pain is often a confusing assessment finding for the nurse practitioner. This symptom appears with notable frequency in diabetic ketoacidosis. Gastric atony and dilation may lead to vomiting and aspiration in the unconscious child. Placement of a nasogastric tube is important while addressing the two urgent issues of evaluation of blood volume and the differential diagnosis of the coma (history of symptoms of nausea, vomiting, thirst, polyuria, weakness, weight loss, and visual disturbances). Kussmaul's breathing commonly occurs (not Cheyne-Stokes) and diaphoresis relates to hypoglycemia. Joint pain is unrelated.

19. **(1)** IDDM usually appears before the age of 30 and is heralded by the trilogy of "Ps"— polydipsia, polyuria, and polyphagia.

20. **(4)** Tight glycemic control is contraindicated in infants <2 years of age and should be instituted with extreme caution in children <7 years of age to avoid injuring the developing brain.

21. **(1)** Infants with hypothyroidism often have an abnormally pitched cry due to lethargy and delayed mental responsiveness. Hypertelorism does not produce an abnormal cry unless accompanied by microcephaly.

# Pharmacology

22. **(3)** Thyroid replacement is lifelong maintenance and should be given as one dose in the morning. Weight loss, diarrhea, and tachycardia are signs of too much thyroid medication.

23. **(3)** A low temperature and pulse, constipation, and fatigue are all signs of hypothyroidism; therefore, the dose of levothyroxine (Synthroid) needs to be increased. Synthroid toxicity would manifest with signs of hyperthyroidism. The constipation is a symptom of hypothyroidism and has nothing to do with the child's fluid intake. Congenital hypothyroidism is a lifelong condition and will require lifelong medication.

24. **(2)** Desmopressin (DDAVP) promotes reabsorption of water in the renal tubules, which can lead to water intoxication. The signs of water intoxication are lethargy, behavioral changes, disorientation, and neuromuscular excitability.

25. **(1)** Insulin injection proportions for the child/adolescent are 2:1 NPH:Regular in the AM and 1:1 in the PM. Changes are made based on blood sugar level done four times a day. The proportion is based on the time periods of insulin activity.

26. **(1)** Lispro (Humalog) is the first analog of human insulin that has several advantages over regular insulin, including a more rapid onset and shorter duration of action. It reaches peak activity in 1–2 hours and has a 4-hour duration, as compared to 6–8 hours for regular insulin. It is convenient for many clients as it can be injected immediately before eating (10–15 minutes). Because it has been on the market only since June 1996, there is no long-term safety profile established and the teratogenicity is unknown. In addition, it is more expensive than insulin and some third-party payers may not reimburse clients.

27. **(2)** Steroid use among adolescent athletes is important to assess. Side effects include reduces physical growth, produces premature epiphyseal closure, causes an increase in breast development in males, decreases testicular size, and produces the appearance of male pattern baldness in men and facial hair in females.

28. **(3)** Acute hypoglycemic episodes in infants must be treated quickly with intravenous administration of glucose at 12–14 mg/kg/min. Diazoxide (Proglycem) can be used as an oral agent to inhibit release of insulin from the pancreas. Although glucagon is a hyperglycemic agent used to elevate blood glucose, it is usually not indicated for infants. Corticosteroids, such as methylprednisolone (Medrol), are of no value in the treatment of hyperinsulinism.

29. **(1)** Growth hormone (usually 0.16–0.24 mg/kg per week, divided into 6–7 doses) is administered by subcutaneous injection into the thigh, buttocks, or abdomen of the child who is still growing (epiphyseal plates are **not** closed or fused).

30. **(3)** Agranulocytosis is a serious reaction that occurs in 1:500 to 1:1000 cases, usually within the first few months of therapy with any type of thionamide (anti-thyroid) medication, i.e., Tapazole, propylthiouracil (PTU). The other three options include minor reactions that subside spontaneously.

# 10

# Musculoskeletal

## Physical Examination & Diagnostic Tests

1. The nurse practitioner places an adolescent in prone position with the knee flexed to 90 degrees. The tibia is firmly opposed to the femur by exerting downward pressure on the foot. The leg is rotated externally and internally. If locking of the knee occurs, this is accurately called a positive:

   1. Drawer sign.
   2. McMurray's test.
   3. Apley's sign.
   4. Bulge sign.

2. What is the name of the sign that occurs when compressing the suprapatellar pouch back against the femur and feeling for fluid entering the spaces?

   1. Drawer sign.
   2. Kernig's sign.
   3. Balloon sign.
   4. Bulge sign.

3. The primary examination techniques to use for assessing the musculoskeletal system are:

   1. Inspection and percussion.
   2. Auscultation and palpation.
   3. Inspection and palpation.
   4. Palpation and percussion.

4. In accurately assessing an adolescent who reports back injury, it is critical to question:

   1. Family history of back problems.
   2. Previous injury.
   3. Personal history of chronic illness.
   4. Mechanism of injury.

5. In the talar tilt test:

   1. The client's foot is held while backward pressure is applied to the tibia. Laxity of the ligament is graded.
   2. The ankle is gently inverted and laxity of the ligament is graded.
   3. The examiner passively inverts, everts, dorsiflexes, and plantar flexes the ankle.
   4. The client actively inverts, everts, dorsiflexes, and plantar flexes the ankle.

115

6. Varus pressure on a knee that is slightly flexed (30 degrees) tests:

    1. Medial collateral ligament stability.

    2. Lateral collateral ligament stability.

    3. Medial cruciate ligament stability.

    4. Lateral meniscus tear.

7. The nurse practitioner is assessing a preadolescent girl for scoliosis. She would:

    1. Have the girl bend at the waist and look for asymmetry in the back and hip area.

    2. Examine the child fully clothed, paying particular attention to the hips and back.

    3. Have the child walk heel-to-toe and observe the gait and pelvis.

    4. Place the child on her back and flex the knees and observe for misalignment.

8. In doing a physical assessment on a newborn, the nurse notes a "hip click." What other findings are associated with this condition?

    1. Shortened quadriceps.

    2. Lateral deviation of patella.

    3. Limited adduction.

    4. Lax hamstrings.

# Disorders

9. A newborn examination reveals inability to dorsiflex either foot, varus position, and a kidney-shaped sole of the foot (when viewed from the bottom). The nurse practitioner's diagnosis is:

    1. Metatarsus varus.

    2. Talipes equinovarus.

    3. Femoral anteversion.

    4. Internal tibial torsion.

10. An adolescent complains of right knee pain immediately after running in track practice. On exam, the knee is warm to touch and a tender, swollen tibial tuberosity is noted. The nurse practitioner suspects:

    1. Osgood-Schlatter's disease.

    2. Rheumatoid arthritis.

    3. Acute tendinitis.

    4. Posttraumatic knee effusion.

11. The nurse practitioner realizes that the most common cause of shoulder pain is:

    1. Frozen shoulder.

    2. Thoracic outlet syndrome.

    3. Impingement syndrome.

    4. Osteochondritis.

12. An adolescent who lifts weights has been diagnosed with a complete rotator cuff tear of the left shoulder. The nurse would expect the client to have difficulty in:

    1. Abducting the left arm.

    2. Supinating the left forearm.

    3. Shrugging the shoulders.

    4. Touching the left hand to the right shoulder.

13. Night-time extremity pain in school-age children that is deep but not present in the joints and is though to be due to inflammation of the muscle bodies in tight fascial sheaths and to periods of high activity is:

    1. Osgood-Schlatter disease.

    2. Patellofemoral stress syndrome.

    3. Growing pains.

    4. Shin splints.

14. The history of a child who may have contacted Lyme disease includes:

    1. Erythematous rash on bridge of nose and cheeks with discoid patches on the trunk.

    2. Immediate development of arthritis symptoms, especially in the knees.

    3. Expanding rash with central clearing occurring within a month of being bitten.

    4. Early symptoms of meningitis and myocarditis.

15. The nurse practitioner is teaching an adolescent with a lower leg cast for a fractured tibia to begin crutch walking. Instructions for assisting the adolescent to walk up the stairs with the crutches would include:

    1. Place both crutches on the upper step and step up with unaffected leg while balancing on crutches.

    2. Position the affected leg on the upper step and use the crutches to move up.

    3. Place the unaffected leg on the upper step and move affected leg and crutches up together.

    4. Position the affected leg and the crutch on the upper step and bring the unaffected leg up with the crutch.

16. The circumstances under which a common injury that can cause a meniscus tear to occur are:

    1. The knee is almost completely extended and the tibia is externally rotated.

    2. An external force is applied that is strong enough to cause external rotation or hyperextension of the knee or a forceful direct blow to the knee.

    3. Valgue or varus pressure on the knee occurs at full extension and at 30 degrees of flexion.

    4. An injury occurs in which the knee is simultaneously twisted and flexed.

17. The nurse practitioner is assessing a radial fracture on a toddler. The fracture is confirmed on x-ray, however there is no bruising, and there is minimal swelling at the fracture site. What condition is important for the nurse practitioner to rule out on this child?

    1. A vascularizing necrosis. *occurs in femur!*

    2. Osteogenesis imperfecta.

    3. Systemic lupus erythematosus.

    4. Carpenter's syndrome. *congenital limb defect*

18. In an event where a knee "gives out," usually associated with trauma, followed by severe pain and effusion and later "locking"

of the knee with pivoting or turning, the client has probably suffered:

    1. Patellofemoral stress syndrome.

    2. Growing pains.

    3. Shin splints.

    4. Patellar subluxation.

19. Quadriceps setting is one exercise recommended for young adults suffering patellofemoral stress syndrome. Teach the client to:

    1. Lie supine on the floor with legs extended. Dorsiflex the foot. Push the thigh into the floor.

    2. Sit on the floor leaning back on the elbows. Flex one knee to 90 degrees and extend one completely. Raise the straight leg until the thigh is parallel to the flexed knee. Hold for 5 seconds. Repeat for opposite leg.

    3. Lie on the floor and flex both knees to about 20 degrees with a rolled-up towel underneath them. Extend one leg and hold for 5 seconds. Repeat for the opposite leg.

    4. Use resistive exercises with an elastic band.

20. In a third-degree ankle strain there is:

    1. Moderate ecchymosis, moderate edema, and a stable joint.

    2. Moderate ecchymosis, moderate edema, and an unstable joint.

    3. Marked ecchymosis, marked edema, and a stable joint.

    4. Marked ecchymosis, marked edema, and an unstable joint.

21. What is the most common cause of "intoeing" in children?

    1. Femoral anteversion.

    2. Metatarsus varus.

    3. Calcaneovalgus.

    4. External tibial torsion.

22. A 15-year-old client presents with complaint of sudden pain and swelling in the knee. He also is complaining of chills and fever. Upon exam, the knee is warm, tender, and swollen with evidence of effusion. The nurse practitioner would:

    1. Splint the affected joint.

    2. Obtain aspiration of synovial fluid from the affected joint.

    3. Initiate treatment with nonsteroidal anti-inflammatory drugs (NSAIDs).

    4. Recommend rest, ice, compresses, and elevation of affected joint.

23. When determining the specific etiology of polyarticular complaints, the clinical clues most helpful for diagnosis are:

    1. Lab identification of antinuclear antibodies (ANAs) and sedimentation rate. ESR

    2. X-ray of affected joints.

    3. Affected joint pattern and presence of or lack of inflammation.

    4. Growth history of client.

24. An adolescent client is being evaluated by the nurse practitioner for knee pain. The client is active in sports in his school but can recall no specific injury to the knee. On exam, the nurse practitioner finds unilateral swelling of the anterior aspect of the tibial tubercle, which is tender. The most likely diagnosis is:

    1. Stress fracture.

    2. Patellar dislocation.

    3. Osgood-Schlatter disease.

    4. Neuman's syndrome.

25. Which of the following is the most accurate statement about juvenile rheumatoid arthritis (JRA)?

    1. Symptoms present with much greater severity than adult rheumatoid arthritis.

    2. Complete remission occurs in three fourths of clients. 3/4 remissions

    3. Over 90% progress to severe joint destruction.

    4. Cytotoxic drugs should be initiated as early as possible in the treatment regimen.

26. In young children, a complaint of hip pain without a history of trauma suggests several differential diagnoses. The diagnosis that is considered a true orthopedic emergency is:

    1. Toxic synovitis of the hip.

    2. Legg-Calvé-Perthes disease.

    3. Increased femoral anteversion.

    4. Avascular necrosis of the femoral head.

27. Primary treatment of joint injury involves:

    1. Rest, ice, compression, and elevation (RICE).

    2. Narcotic pain control and x-ray.

    3. Specialist referral and magnetic resonance imaging.

    4. NSAIDs and exercise.

28. The most common complaint in a client with back injury who had cauda equina syndrome, a surgical emergency, is:

    1. Urinary retention.

    2. Numbness below the level of injury.

    3. Weakness in the lower extremities.

    4. Pain.

29. Children with JRA must be screened regularly for:

    1. Ulcerative colitis.

    2. Iridocyclitis. (Uveitis)

    3. Diabetes mellitus.

    4. Adrenal insufficiency.

30. An adolescent twisted his knee while skateboarding. He complains of knee pain and also states that, in the past few weeks, his knee has "locked up" a couple of times. Upon examination, a positive McMurray's test is elicited. This is consistent with a diagnosis of:

    1. Anterior cruciate ligament tear.

2. Dislocated patella.

3. Medial meniscus tear.

4. Chondromalacia patella.

31. Differentiation between structural and functional scoliosis can be done by placing the child in Adams' position. In this position:

    1. Structural disappears and functional is enhanced.

    2. Persistent functional scoliosis is indicated.

    3. Functional disappears and structural is enhanced.

    4. Curves >10 degrees are indicated.

32. A 2-month-old child is in the clinic for a well-child examination. The mother is concerned that his feet are crooked and turn inward. Physical exam reveals feet deviate inward and heel position is dorsiflexed in valgus when examined from behind; no other abnormalities are noted. The nurse practitioner diagnoses this as:

    1. Metatarsus valgus.

    2. Talipes equinovarus.

    3. Calcaneovalgus.

    4. Congenital clubfoot.

33. A male child with pectis excavatum and an associated scoliosis should be evaluated for:

    1. Pulmonary dysfunction.

    2. Cardiac compromise.

    3. Marfan syndrome.

    4. Joint deformities.

34. The nurse practitioner understands that a Salter IV fracture:

    1. Does not involve the growth plate and usually presents with tenderness over the growth plate.

    2. Is the most common injury where a fragment of the metaphyseal bone separates from the epiphysis.

    3. Rarely occurs and involves a compression of the growth plate, leading to disturbed bone growth.

    4. Involves a fracture across the growth plate that injures both the epiphysis and the metaphysis.

35. The nurse practitioner understands that transient subluxation of the proximal radial head is often called:

    1. Toddler's fracture.

    2. Nursemaid's elbow.

    3. Boxer's subluxation.

    4. Adams' subluxation.

36. A mother states that her newborn has a "fractured collarbone." Physical exam reveals:

    1. Limited abduction of the arm on the unaffected side.

    2. Decreased arm movement on the affected side.

    3. Lack of crepitus and edema.

    4. Increased laxity of the muscles.

# Pharmacology

37. Medications used in the treatment of juvenile arthritis include:

    1. Ibuprofen (Motrin, Advil) only.

    2. Oral corticosteroids (prednisone, methylprednisolone).

    3. Azathioprine (Imuran), cyclophosphamide (Cytoxan), and chlorambucil (Leukeran).

    4. Aspirin, hydroxychloroquine (Plaquenil), and gold sodium thimalate (Myochyrsine).

38. Gold compounds are contraindicated in clients with all of the following **except**:

    1. Renal disease.

    2. Hepatic disease.

    3. Rheumatoid arthritis.

    4. Blood dyscrasia.

39. A child has been on hydroxychloroquine (Plaquenil) for 6 months. This was the medication of choice for her severe juvenile rheumatoid arthritis. The nurse practitioner would expect all of the following **except**:

    1. An ophthalmology examination is required every 6 months.

    2. The mother notices that the child's hair appears bleached and thinning.

    3. Effects of the medication are slow acting and take weeks to achieve therapeutic levels.

    4. Coagulation studies, electrolytes, and complete blood count are performed every week.

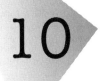

# 10  Answers & Rationales

## Physical Examination & Diagnostic Tests

1. **(3)** Apley's sign, locking of the knee or the sound of clicks and pain, may indicate a loose body, such as torn cartilage. This test is performed to detect a torn meniscus. The drawer sign tests the collateral ligaments with the client in a sitting and lying position, not prone. The McMurray's test is a test for medial meniscus injury. In this test, the knee is fully flexed and the tibia is externally rotated. Varus pressure is applied to the knee while it is extended. To test for medial meniscus tear, the test is performed while applying valgus pressure to the knee.

2. **(3)** The balloon sign occurs in instances when considerable fluid is in the suprapatellar pouch; ballottement of the patella may be possible. The bulge sign is for testing fluid in the knee joint and is elicited with the knee extended by applying pressure to the medial aspect of the knee and watching for a bulge or fluid wave. A patellar tap suggests fluid in the knee as the patella clicks against the femur. The drawer sign tests the collateral ligaments with the client in a sitting and lying position. Kernig's sign, a sign of meningeal irritation, is the inability to extend the lower leg when that leg is flexed at the hip; there may also be resistance or pain during elicitation of the sign.

3. **(3)** The musculoskeletal system is examined by visual inspection and palpation of bones, joints, and surrounding muscular tissue. Percussion is generally not done, and auscultation is not appropriate to the system being examined.

4. **(4)** A thorough history is very important in assessing any client with injury, but, in the event of a back injury, the mechanism of injury will provide the greatest clue as to the extent of injury and the proper path to take in diagnosis and treatment.

5. **(2)** Gentle inversion of the affected ankle in an ankle injury is compared with the unaffected ankle in the talar tilt test. Anterior ankle stability is tested in the anterior drawer test, in which the tibia is grasped by one of the examiner's hands while the heel is firmly grasped and backward pressure is applied to the tibia with the examiner's other hand. In passive range of motion, the examiner inverts, everts, dorsiflexes, and plantar flexes the foot and ankle. The client puts the foot and ankle through complete range of motion in active range of motion.

6. **(2)** Varus pressure on a slightly flexed knee tests for lateral collateral ligament stability. Valgus pressure tests for medial collateral ligament stability. Cruciate ligaments are tested with the anterior drawer test. The McMurray's test is a test for medial meniscus injury. In this test, the knee is fully flexed and the tibia is externally rotated. Varus pressure is applied to the knee while it is extended. To test for medial meniscus tear, the test is performed while applying valgus pressure to the knee.

7. **(1)** The child should remove her shirt (leave on bra or swimsuit top) and bend at the waist. The nurse should examine for uneven hips and shoulders.

8. **(4)** Typical findings include Ortolani's (hip click) sign, limited abduction, shortening of the extremity on the affected side, and asymmetrical gluteal folds. The lax hamstrings allow for full extension of the hip when the knee is fully flexed. Tight hip abductors in the neonatal period are not a sign of congenital hip dislocation.

# Disorders

9. **(2)** These are classic findings for talipes equinovarus. In metatarsus varus the foot is easily dorsiflexed. Femoral anteversion is the cause of intoeing. Internal tibial torsion (physiologic bowing of lower extremities) is a normal finding in the newborn.

10. **(1)** Osgood-Schlatter's disease (tibial tubercle apophysitis) is characterized by a painful, self-limiting tibial tubercle swelling that leads to knee pain, especially during periods of rapid growth. Extension of the knee against resistance or application of pressure over the tibial tubercle aggravates the pain. Pain worsens with activity and lessens with rest.

11. **(3)** Impingement syndrome is usually caused by rotator cuff tendinitis, which occurs when internal/external rotation is impaired. Frozen shoulder can occur after a rotator cuff injury, especially if a sling is used for a prolonged period of time. Osteochondritis dessecans is a condition where the femoral condyle is damaged and can break free in the knee joint.

12. **(1)** With a complete rotator cuff tear (rupture of the supraspinatus tendon), the client would have difficulty abducting the arm and impaired internal/external rotation. Touching the hand to the opposite shoulder is adduction.

13. **(3)** Growing pains usually occur at night and resolve by morning. The pain is deep and does not involve the joints. Osgood-Schlatter disease is due to degeneration of the tibial tubercle due to overuse and a rapid growth spurt. Pain and swelling occur over the tibial tubercle. Symptoms are exacerbated by activities that involve the quadriceps muscle. Another form of overuse syndrome is patellofemoral stress syndrome. Pain of a dull, aching quality is present in the knee, sometimes with clicking. Long periods of sitting or activities that involve knee flexion as well as compression of the patella in the groove cause increased pain. In shin splints, inflammation of muscles along the medial shaft of the tibia is due to overuse and causes aching pain. Rest improves the pain. Improper warm-up exercises or a lot of exercise by an unconditioned person, especially in unsuitable shoes, can lead to this pain.

14. **(3)** Option #1 describes the malar or "butterfly" rash of systemic lupus erythematosus. The arthritis symptoms and other complications (meningitis and myocarditis) occur later in the disease process, especially if child is not treated with antibiotics (usually tetracycline, doxycycline, or amoxicillin).

15. **(3)** The unaffected leg goes up the step first; then the crutches and affected leg follow. This allows for stability and weight-bearing on the unaffected leg, with the crutches supporting the affected leg.

16. **(4)** A client who sustained a meniscal tear can usually recall a twisting injury of the knee followed by pain and effusion over the joint line. A strong force or injury that causes external rotation or hyperextension of the knee is a common mechanism of collateral or cruciate ligament injuries. A test for stability of the knee joint involves applying medial and lateral pressure to the knee during full extension and flexion of 30 degrees.

17. **(2)** Osteogenesis imperfecta is referred to as the "brittle bone disease" and is the most common genetic disorder of the bone in children. It is a group of hereditary diseases characterized by excess bone fragility with increase tendency to fracture. Carpenter's syndrome is a congenital limb defect, and a vascularizing necrosis occurs in the femur.

18. **(4)** At the time a patellar subluxation occurs, a traumatic event causes the knee to

"give out" and the patella is laterally displaced. Severe pain and an effusion result. Subsequent to the injury, the client will notice a locking sensation in the knee with pivoting or turning. A form of overuse syndrome is patellofemoral stress syndrome. Pain of a dull, aching quality is present in the knee, sometimes with clicking. Long periods of sitting or activities that involve knee flexion as well as compression of the patella in the groove cause increased pain. Growing pains usually occur at night and resolve by morning. The pain is deep and does not involve the joints. In shin splints, inflammation of muscles along the medial shaft of the tibia due to overuse causes aching pain. Rest improves the pain. Improper warm-up exercises or a lot of exercise by an unconditioned person, especially in unsuitable shoes, can lead to this pain.

19. **(1)** In quadriceps setting, with the foot dorsiflexed, the thigh is pressed down against the floor and held for 5 seconds. The straight leg raise involves lifting an extended leg while sitting on the floor and leaning back on the elbows with the opposite leg flexed to 90 degrees. A terminal arc extension requires that the client lie on the floor supine with extended legs flexed to 20 degrees over a rolled-up towel. The client then extends one leg and holds for 5 seconds. The exercise is repeated for the opposite leg. All of the above exercises can be used to stretch and strengthen the quadriceps muscles in those suffering from patellofemoral stress syndrome, however, Option #1 describes typical "quadriceps setting." Resistive exercises with an elastic band are general exercises that can be done with the extremities.

20. **(4)** A third-degree strain is a complete tear of the ligament resulting in marked edema, ecchymosis, and pain and an unstable joint.

21. **(1)** Femoral anteversion is the most common cause of intoeing in children. This normally decreases as the child grows, with about 80–90% of the cases resolving to a normal range.

22. **(2)** Symptoms are indicative of septic arthritis, which is a medical emergency; if not treated promptly, the joint may be destroyed. Examination of the joint fluid is the single most important diagnostic test. Other choices may provide some symptomatic relief, but the first goal of treatment is to determine if the joint is septic.

23. **(3)** When developing differential diagnosis, the history and physical exam will help narrow the differentiation. Other procedures are important in completing the evaluation, but the most important information is the pattern of joints affected and whether it is inflammatory or noninflammatory disease.

24. **(3)** Osgood-Schlatter disease is common in late childhood and adolescence. The likelihood increases in clients who are involved in strenuous activity, especially that involving the quadriceps muscle. The usual treatment is NSAIDs and rest.

25. **(2)** Most clients do not have disease persistent into adulthood. JRA symptoms present very similar to adult arthritis. Most disease activity diminishes with age; although some clients do have some residual joint damage, it is not this high a percentage. Aspirin is the treatment of choice; cytotoxic drugs are reserved for clients who have failed other therapy.

26. **(4)** Toxic synovitis and increased femoral anteversion, while causing pain, are not bone threatening. Legg-Calvé-Perthes disease results in necrosis of the proximal femoral epiphysis; however, there is later revascularization. Avascular necrosis results in death of the femoral head without revascularization.

27. **(1)** The RICE principle is used for initial treatment: **R**est, **I**ce, **C**ompression, and **E**levation. All other treatments mentioned may be appropriate, but not as the primary treatment.

28. **(1)** Although all of the above symptoms may be associated with cauda equina syndrome, urinary retention is the most important clue to the immediate need for surgery.

29. **(2)** Development of iridocyclitis may be insidious and asymptomatic, and if left untreated may cause blindness. Although children may develop any of these other diseases, there is no correlation with JRA.

30. **(3)** A positive McMurray's test (palpable click and pain when rotating the foot laterally and extending the leg), along with the symptoms mentioned, is indicative of a medial meniscus tear. The drawer test evaluates for anterior cruciate ligament tears (i.e., knee flexed with foot on table; sit on foot and grasp both sides of tibia at the knee; pull tibia forward; abnormal if movement of tibia away from the joint).

31. **(3)** In Adams' position (forward bending, arms loose at side, thumbs hooked together), true scoliosis (structural) is demonstrated (by an elevated rib hump), whereas the functional type related to other conditions is not apparent. Persistent functional scoliosis can eventually become structural.

32. **(3)** This is a common problem associated with abnormal or positional confinement in utero. Inspection reveals a banana-shaped sole (lateral deviation).

33. **(3)** Pectus excavatum can affect cardiopulmonary function but, when associated with scoliosis, the child should be evaluated for Marfan syndrome.

34. **(4)** The Salter-Harris classification system for fractures is a way to describe injury to the growth plate. Option #4 describes a Salter IV fracture, which must be perfectly aligned to protect growth potential. Option #1 describes a Salter I fracture. Option #2 describes a Salter II. Option #3 describes a Salter V.

35. **(2)** This common dislocation is called "nursemaid's elbow." It is caused by inadvertent pulling or yanking of a child's arm, often by the parent or caretaker. Usually, it occurs in children ages 1–4. The child often refuses to move the arm and keeps it flexed and pronated. A toddler's fracture is frequently referred to as a spiral fracture of the tibia.

36. **(2)** Fractured clavicles can occur throughout childhood and have an increased incidence during vaginal deliveries, especially if the infant is large for gestational age or there is a difficult delivery. There usually is crepitus and swelling at the fracture site.

# Pharmacology

37. **(4)** NSAIDs, along with the medications listed in Option #4, are the common medications used to treat juvenile arthritis. Oral steroids (Option #2) are contraindicated, and intra-articular injection may be used but can lead to cartilage and bone necrosis with repeated injections. Use of the drugs listed in Option #3 is controversial.

38. **(3)** Gold is indicated for treatment of rheumatoid arthritis and is contraindicated in the presence of the other diseases mentioned.

39. **(4)** Visual complications are associated with Plaquenil; therefore, the child should be monitored by an ophthalmologist every 6 months. Other side effects include bleaching and loss of hair, anorexia, abdominal discomfort, and neuromuscular weakness. Option #4 is not associated with this medication.

# Neurology

## Physical Examination & Diagnostic Tests

1. To determine cerebellar functioning in the older pediatric client, the practitioner evaluates:

   1. Ability of the client to balance on one foot, then the other.

   2. Discriminatory sensation between two familiar objects.

   3. Ability to recall names of three U.S. presidents.

   4. Range of motion and ability to move extremities.

2. What is considered a "soft" neurologic (or equivocal) sign?

   1. Positive Babinski's reflex in an adult.

   2. Mirroring hand movements of the extremities.

   3. Brudzinski's sign.

   4. Kernig's sign.

3. A child is having problems controlling her seizures. Prior to electroencephalography

(EEG), the nurse practitioner explains to the child and parents that:

   1. This test will cause some discomfort and she will be given a sedative before the test.

   2. It will be important for her to take her regular dose of fluoxetine (Prozac) and phenytoin Dilantin) prior to the test.

   3. The procedure is painless and she will not be in any discomfort or experience electrical shock during the procedure.

   4. After the test, she will be on bed rest for 8 hours and will be given full liquids for 12 hours.

4. Which cranial nerve is being tested when the nurse practitioner asks the child to raise her eyebrows, smile, frown, or puff out her cheeks?

   1. Hypoglossal nerve.

   2. Acoustic nerve.

   3. Glossopharyngeal nerve.

   4. Facial nerve.

*→ grandmal sz = tonn-clonic sz/epilepsy*
*shaky*

5. The nurse practitioner notes an absent knee jerk reflex in a healthy child. What might the nurse practitioner ask the child to do?

   1. Lift both arms above the head and count to 5 slowly as reflex is tested.

   2. Raise both legs slowly and then lower and immediately test for the reflex.

   3. Clench both hands together and pull while the reflex is tested.

   4. Close eyes and hold breath while examiner tests for the reflex.

6. The nurse practitioner gently flexes a child's neck in the direction of the chin touching the chest. If there is pain and resistance to the flexion and the hips and knees flex at the same time, the nurse practitioner accurately describes this finding as:

   1. Phalen's sign.

   2. Romberg's sign.

   3. Kernig's sign

   4. Brudzinski's sign.

7. To test the cremasteric reflex, the nurse practitioner would:

   1. Stroke the upper inner thigh.

   2. Stimulate the skin in the perianal area.

   3. Stroke the skin toward the umbilicus.

   4. Strike the Achilles tendon.

8. To begin an assessment of cerebral function in a school-age child, the nurse practitioner might start out with which of the following questions?

   1. "Have you noticed a change in your ability to remember things?"

   2. "Have you noticed any change in your sense of smell?"

   3. "Do you have any problems with your balance?"

   4. "Do you have any numbness or tingling in your fingers?"

9. Which statement is correct regarding classification of seizures in pediatrics?

   1. Clonic seizures, repetitive stiffening and contracting, are long in duration and rarely occur in childhood.

   2. Tonic seizures, characterized by violent shaking, were previously called grand mal. *non shaky*

   3. Febrile seizures occur in young children between the ages of 3 months and 5 years.

   4. Infantile spasms are characterized by rapid tonic–clonic movements, lasting several minutes.

## Disorders

10. A tool that the nurse practitioner might use to further diagnose headaches is:

    1. A headache diary kept by the child and family.

    2. The child's most recent report card.

    3. A Connor Scale completed by parents and teachers.

    4. A personality evaluation from the school psychologist.

11. An adolescent has a history of injury at the level of the fifth thoracic vertebra (T5) and his condition has stabilized. The nurse practitioner understands that, with this level of injury, the adolescent is most likely not going to be able to:

    1. Perform coordinated movements with his hands, such as writing.

    2. Achieve lower body strength and coordination for walking.

    3. Have upper body strength adequate enough to drive a car.

    4. Maintain upper body coordination required to feed himself.

12. The nurse practitioner understands that the early signs that suggest cerebral palsy are:

    1. Difficulty feeding.

    2. Meningitis.

3. Profound hypotonicity.

4. Symmetrical diminished tonic neck reflex.

13. A teenage client is admitted to a rural clinic after a diving accident. The nurse practitioner suspects a spinal cord injury at cervical level 5 (C5). While awaiting emergency transport services, the nurse practitioner assesses for the development of complications by:

1. Checking for voluntary movement of extremities and sensation below level of injury.

2. Assessing breath sounds and evaluating movement of diaphragm with respirations.

3. Maintaining cervical flexion to facilitate airway until cervical traction is initiated.

4. Beginning neurologic checks with careful documentation of location of pain sensations.

14. Epidemic meningococcal meningitis occurs rarely. This control is due to:

1. Use of active immunization.

2. Lower community carrier rates.

3. Improved socioeconomic conditions.

4. Earlier detection and recognition of outbreaks.

15. The nurse practitioner is assessing a young male child. What observations would indicate a positive Gower's sign?

1. The use of both hands to brace his legs as he raises himself to a standing position.

2. Sensory loss of bladder control resulting in a neurogenic bladder.

3. The inability to extend his legs fully when lying supine.

4. Bilateral loss of ability to move lower extremities.

16. In infants, especially preterm infants, seizures can present as:

1. Coughing spells.

2. Poor feeding.

3. Awake apnea.

4. Regurgitation.

17. An older child is brought to the clinic by his mother. There is unilateral ptosis, and the child complains of double vision. On examination there is weakness noted in extraocular movements. What diagnostic test would assist to identify this condition?

1. Tensilon test.

2. Cerebral spinal fluid analysis.

3. Peripheral nerve conduction time studies.

4. Intraocular pressure and examination of fundal fields.

18. Which is a pathophysiologic reason for a headache?

1. Vascular constriction of the middle meningeal artery.

2. Muscle strain.

3. Dysregulation of the ascending brain stem serotonergic system.

4. Inflammation of the scalp.

19. What viral illnesses are most frequently associated with the development of Reye's syndrome?

1. Respiratory infections, varicella, diarrhea.

2. Rubella, juvenile arthritis, systemic lupus erythematosus.

3. Encephalitis, tuberculosis, respiratory infections.

4. Varicella, meningitis, Guillain-Barré.

20. A 3-week-old infant has been diagnosed with bacterial meningitis. The nurse practitioner is aware that the most common causative organism is:

1. *Streptococcus pyogenes.*

2. *Streptococcus pneumoniae.*

3. *Neisseria meningitidis.*

4. Group B streptococcus.

21. The nurse practitioner is caring for a 10-year-old child with meningitis. To assess for the presence of nuchal rigidity, the nurse practitioner would:

    1. Have the child bend forward at the waist and observe the line of the spine.

    2. Place her hand on the child's forehead and ask the child to press against her hand with his head.

    3. With the child relaxed, attempt to move the child's head from side to side.

    4. Place her hand on the back of the child's head and assist the child to put his chin on his chest.

22. A young adolescent is accompanied to the clinic by her mother, who states that the school reports that the girl stares off into space a lot and does not seem to pay attention during these brief periods, which typically last 1–3 minutes. The neurologic exam is within normal limits. The nurse practitioner suspects:

    1. Grand mal seizure.

    2. Complex partial seizure.

    3. Absence seizure.

    4. Simple partial seizure.

23. A child is admitted to the rural clinic following a car accident in which she sustained a closed head injury and fractured femur. The child is very lethargic and follows commands very slowly, and her pupils are equal and reactive. The child is to be transferred to a hospital by air ambulance. In evaluating significant changes in her condition, the nurse practitioner would be most concerned with which finding?

    1. Urine output is below 30 cc/hr.

    2. Complaints of a headache are noted in the frontal area.

    3. She is unable to move her right arm and leg.

    4. Vital signs are BP 130/50, pulse 70.

24. A parent whose son was recently diagnosed with Tourette's syndrome asks the nurse practitioner about the condition. The nurse practitioner understands that:

    1. Tourette's syndrome is commonly treated with antianxiety agents, such as diazepam (Valium).

    2. Tics occur many times throughout the day and they change over time.

    3. Children rarely will have attention deficit hyperactivity disorder (ADHD) in conjunction with Tourette's syndrome.

    4. Tics are commonly neuromuscular, such as facial grimacing, tongue protruding, and neck twitching; rarely are the tics vocal.

25. A 3-year-old child presents to the nurse practitioner with a history of hospitalization at 18 months for bacterial meningitis. The nurse practitioner would want to be sure to include:

    1. Vision testing.

    2. Hearing testing.

    3. Lumbar puncture.

    4. Electrocardiogram.

26. Which is considered a likely cause of seizures in adolescents and young adults?

    1. Congenital abnormalities and metabolic disturbances.

    2. Metabolic disorders, central nervous system infection, and fever.

    3. Idiopathic seizures, trauma, and substance abuse.

    4. Trauma, malignant tumor, and cerebral vascular accident.

27. A child presents with a history of a purpuric rash with a centrifugal distribution and a fever. The nurse practitioner who examines this child should be highly suspicious of:

    1. Rubella.

    2. Lyme disease.

    3. Meningococcemia.

    4. Roseola.

28. The mother of a 5-year-old boy brings him to the clinic with complaints that he is

"acting funny." She states there are short periods of time when he does not respond to her, he does not fall, then he suddenly responds and acts as if nothing has happened. The nurse would initially evaluate the child further for the presence of:

1. Petit mal or absence seizures.

2. Attention deficit disorder.

3. Prodrome prior to episode.

4. Avoidance disorder of childhood.

29. The nurse practitioner observes a seizure in a 3-year-old. There is involvement of the right arm, and the activity spreads to involve all of the muscles on the right side of the body. There was transient paralysis of the right side after the seizure. What is the classification of this type of seizure?

1. Generalized tonic-clonic seizure.

2. Complex partial seizure.

3. Atonic absence seizure.

4. Simple partial seizure.

30. The nurse practitioner understands that the general criterion for diagnosis of status epilepticus is:

1. Tonic-clonic seizures with a 10 minute duration.

2. Any seizure that continues for 30 minutes.

3. Intermittent seizures lasting 5 minutes in duration where the person regains partial consciousness between the episodes.

4. Intermittent myoclonic seizures lasting 15 minutes where the person does not regain consciousness between the episodes.

31. The nurse practitioner knows that the American Academy of Pediatrics recommends chemoprophylaxis for meningococcal disease for:

1. All household, day care, or preschool contacts or anyone directly exposed to the child's secretions.

2. Only household contacts.

3. Anyone who exhibits symptoms within 1 week of the index case.

4. Only those close contacts who are immunocompromised.

32. An 18-month-old infant just experienced a first febrile seizure with a concurrent diagnosis of otitis media. The nurse practitioner will teach the child's mother to:

1. Give anticonvulsant medication every day, as ordered by the neurologist.

2. Treat fevers aggressively in the future.

3. Give anticonvulsant medication at the first sign of a febrile illness.

4. Take the child to the clinic for evaluation if the temperature is above 100°F (rectally).

33. A 1-month-old infant comes to the nurse practitioner's office with a rectal temp of 102.5°F for 12 hours. The temperature does come down with acetaminophen (Tylenol). On physical exam, the baby is fussy, but no specific focus of infection is found. Appropriate action for the nurse practitioner includes:

1. Send baby home with instructions for mother to feed Pedialyte and return to the office in 24 hours for re-evaluation.

2. Instruct mother to use ibuprofen (Advil) for the temperature.

3. Prescribe an antibiotic to cover potential infections.

4. Consult with a pediatrician to arrange for further evaluation.

34. A child with a migraine headache is most likely to complain of pain in:

1. The frontal area of the head.

2. The occipital area of the head.

3. The temporal area of the head.

4. Multiple areas of the head.

35. Which condition is not included in the differential diagnosis of seizure?

    1. Night terrors.

    2. Breathholding or hysteria.

    3. Cerebral vascular disease.

    4. Syncope.

36. Characteristics of headaches that would not suggest increased intracranial pressure include headaches that:

    1. Wake the child up.

    2. Occur in the early morning.

    3. Are accompanied by vomiting without nausea.

    4. Occur several times a week in the afternoon.

# Pharmacology

37. A child is on antiepileptic medication. The nurse practitioner understands that antiepileptic medication:

    1. Must be taken indefinitely.

    2. Is usually discontinued after 4 years of no seizure activity, following an EEG test to confirm lack of seizure activity.

    3. Is usually given in combination with other antiepileptics or sedatives to reduce the seizure threshold.

    4. Must be given to all children who experience a seizure.

38. During a physical exam of a child diagnosed with chronic recurrent seizures who is receiving antiepileptic medication, the nurse practitioner notes hyperplasia of the gums. The nurse understands that hyperplasia of the gums is:

    1. An unusual side effect of phenobarbital.

    2. A common side effect of phenytoin.

    3. A common occurrence with chronic recurrent seizures.

    4. Due to poor oral hygiene.

39. Infantile spasms are usually treated with:

    1. Phenytoin (Dilantin).

    2. Phenobarbital (Luminal).

    3. Adrenocorticotropic hormone (ACTH).

    4. Carbamazepine (Tegretol).

40. The nurse practitioner understands the following about phenobarbital (Luminal) use in children.

    1. Paradoxical central nervous system (CNS) hyperactivity or nervousness may occur.

    2. It can be safely used for the treatment of insomnia and night terrors.

    3. Frequent side effects are decreased attention span and discoloration of urine.

    4. Gingival hyperplasia occurs with long-term usage.

# 11 Answers & Rationales

## Physical Examination & Diagnostic Tests

1. **(1)** The cerebellar area controls gross motor movements and balance, as well as fine motor movements of upper and lower extremities. Discriminatory sensations tests the sensory system, and a remote memory test is a mental status examination involving the cerebral cortex.

2. **(2)** Soft neurologic signs involve slight deviations of the central nervous system (CNS) that are present occasionally or inconsistently. Examples are short attention span, clumsiness, frequent falling (disturbances of gait), hyperkinesis, left-handedness but right-footedness, language disturbances, ansacoria, and mirroring movements of the extremities (when one hand performs, the other is in motion also). The other three options indicate CNS problems that occur consistently (i.e., Brudzinski's and Kernig's signs indicate meningeal irritation; a positive Babinski's reflex in an adult may indicate an upper motor lesion in the corticospinal tract).

3. **(3)** The procedure is painless, and there is no danger of electrical shock. No anticonvulsants, antidepressants, stimulants (caffeine, tobacco), or alcohol should be taken. There is no restriction on movement or diet after the procedure.

4. **(4)** The facial nerve is tested by facial movement, taste, sensation, and corneal reflex. The hypoglossal nerve is tested by the client sticking out his tongue. The acoustic nerve is tested by a hearing test. The glossopharyngeal nerve is tested by taste, gag reflex, and giving the client a drink and asking him to swallow.

5. **(3)** Augmentation of the knee jerk reflex can be obtained by having the child isometrically tense muscles not directly involved with the reflex arc being tested. This is called Jendrassik's maneuver.

6. **(4)** This describes Brudzinski's sign. Phalen's sign is elicited in carpal tunnel syndrome. Romberg's test is done to assess gross swaying by asking the client to stand with feet together and eyes closed for 5 seconds. Kernig's sign (inability to extend the lower leg when the leg is flexed at the hip, or resistance or pain during the process) along with Brudzinski's sign indicate meningeal irritation and should be further evaluated.

7. **(1)** Stroking the upper thigh tests for the cremasteric reflex. Stimulating the skin in the perianal area tests the anal reflex. Stroking the skin toward the umbilicus stimulates the abdominal reflex. Striking the Achilles tendon tests the Achilles reflex. The cremasteric, anal, and abdominal reflexes are superficial reflexes, whereas the Achilles reflex is a deep tendon reflex.

8. **(1)** Cerebral function is demonstrated by thinking, remembering and other cognitive skills. Sense of smell is controlled by the olfactory cranial nerve. Balance is controlled by cerebellar function. Numbness or tingling would be indicative of local nerve involvement.

9. **(3)** Febrile seizures occur in young children between the ages of 3 months and 5 years. They are typically tonic–clonic-type seizures of brief duration and occur due to high fever. Clonic seizures are repetitive jerks or shaking of the body that are brief in duration but can last a few minutes, and occur in early in childhood. Tonic seizures are rapid, violent muscular contractions or stiffening (not shaking) of the body. The tonic–clonic seizure was previously called the grand mal seizure. Infantile spasms (West's syndrome) occur between the ages of 3 months and 1 year and are characterized by flexor, extensor, and mixed-type spasms; they are repetitive, last for seconds at a time, and appear in clusters that can last 10–15 minutes at a time.

## Disorders

10. **(1)** A headache diary can be very useful to identify when the headaches occur, what the child is doing at the onset, what measures afford relief, and the child's and parent's participation in the process of identifying headaches and promoting relief. Pain can also be classified on a numerical scale of 1–10 or using one of the preschool pain scales for the younger child. The Connor Scale, when completed by parents and teachers, is useful in evaluating the child with attention deficit disorder (ADD) with or without hyperactivity (ADHD). The child's school performance, as recorded on report cards and psychologist's evaluations, may enhance the diagnostic picture but is not particularly helpful in making the diagnosis of headaches.

11. **(2)** T5 injuries do not affect the coordination or capacity of the upper body, arms and hands; the lower body is paralyzed. The adolescent should be able to do all of the activities listed except walk.

12. **(1)** Early signs of cerebral palsy include difficulty feeding often due to tongue thrusting, tonic bite, or oral hypersensitivity. In addition, irritability, delayed milestones such as head control, exaggerated or persistent infantile reflexes, such as asymmetrical tonic neck response, hyperreflexia, and asymmetry may be seen.

13. **(2)** At this level of injury (C5), the intercostal muscles and diaphragm can be affected and the client will have respiratory compromise. Airway maintenance and avoiding flexion of the neck are critical.

14. **(3)** Undoubtedly, improved sanitary and socioeconomic conditions have led to the marked reduction in the number of cases of epidemic meningitis. There is no research to support increased cases in communities with higher carrier numbers.

15. **(1)** Gower's sign is classic in muscular dystrophy. The child or adolescent cannot move himself into the standing position without bracing his legs with his hands.

16. **(3)** While it is important to investigate all episodes of apnea in infants, premature infants may not exhibit the typical tonic–clonic-type seizures but may have awake apnea.

17. **(1)** The Tensilon test is used to assist to identify myasthenia gravis. In myasthenia gravis clients there is an immediate but brief improvement in the muscle tone when the medications are injected. Electrodiagnostic evaluation of muscle response will be more definitive of myasthenia gravis.

18. **(3)** Stimulation of pain-sensitive structures, vessel and meningeal inflammation, vasodilation, severe muscle contraction in the head and neck area, and dysregulation of the ascending brain stem serotonergic system are causes for headaches.

19. **(1)** These are the three conditions most frequently associated with the development of Reye's syndrome.

20. **(4)** The most common cause of bacterial meningitis in the first month of life is the Group B streptococcus. *Streptococcus pneumoniae* and *Neisseria meningitidis* are usually associated with meningitis after the

age of 1 month in areas where the conjugate *Haemophilus influenzae* type B (Hib) vaccines are used.

21. **(4)** Nuchal rigidity is a stiff neck; the child cannot move his head forward and cannot bring his chin in contact with his chest. Movement of the head from side to side does not elicit nuchal rigidity.

22. **(3)** This accurately fits the description of a petit mal or absence seizure, which is a type of generalized seizure that begins in childhood and usually ends in early adulthood (30s). There is usually impairment of consciousness, automatic symptoms, and mild tonic–clonic symptoms. Classically, "the staring off into space" is the reporting symptom.

23. **(4)** Increase in pulse pressure and decrease in pulse rate are indications of increasing cerebral edema and intracranial pressure and would necessitate immediate intervention. A child's urine output should be between 20 and 30 ml/hr. The loss of movement on one side of the body would be very uncommon in a child with a head injury.

24. **(2)** Tourette's syndrome is a hereditary, chronic neuromuscular disorder consisting of various motor and vocal tics. Tics are sudden, involuntary, brief, repetitive motor movements that often begin in childhood and change over time. Neuroleptic drugs, such as haloperidol (Haldol), are the medications of choice. ADHD frequently occurs concomitantly with Tourette's syndrome.

25. **(2)** It would be most important to do a formal hearing acuity test on a child with a history of bacterial meningitis due to the use of ototoxic medications used to treat the disease. A vision test should be done on all children but is not specific for a child with a history of meningitis. A lumbar puncture or electrocardiogram would not be appropriate.

26. **(3)** The most likely causes of seizures in adolescents are idiopathic disease, trauma, and substance abuse. Congenital abnormalities are the likely cause of seizures in newborns. In children <6 years old, metabolic causes, central nervous system infection, or fever can cause seizures.

27. **(3)** The most common finding in children with meningococcemia (71%) is fever and a purpuric rash. The rashes of rubella, Lyme disease, and roseola are finer, and none of these problems is life threatening, as is meningococcemia, making it a "do not miss" diagnosis.

28. **(1)** The description is that of a petit or absence seizure. The client should have a neurologic work-up to determine the cause of the seizures. There is no prodrome or aura in absence seizures.

29. **(4)** Simple partial seizures (Jacksonian) are brief and are characterized by focal motor activity, especially on one side of the body. Transient paralysis may follow simple partial seizures in young children.

30. **(2)** Any seizure that continues for 30 minutes, or intermittent seizures lasting for 30 minutes in which the person does not regain consciousness between the episodes is the most commonly accepted criterion for status epilepticus.

31. **(1)** This is the current recommendation of the American Academy of Pediatrics. Studies have demonstrated that these contacts have a rate of infection approximately 100–800 times that of the general population. In addition, 50% of the secondary cases occur within 5 days of the index case, and 70% within 1 week. Rifampin is 90% effective in eliminating carriage of the meningococcus from the nasopharynx. The dose is 10 mg/kg (maximum adult dose is 600 mg) q12h for 2 days for children over 1 month of age and 5 mg/kg q12h for 2 days for infants less than 1 month of age.

32. **(2)** Healthy infants and children who experience a simple febrile seizure (lasts less than 25 minutes and does not recur within 24 hours) are not usually placed on anticonvulsant medication. Instead, parents are taught to treat fevers aggressively in future illnesses in an attempt to prevent subsequent seizures.

33. **(4)** Sepsis must be considered as a possible diagnosis in a febrile infant less than 2 months of age with no focus of infection noted. This child could be critically ill in 24 hours upon re-evaluation. Ibuprofen is not recommended in children <6 months of age. Prescribing an antibiotic without an identified infection can result in a partially treated meningitis or in inaccurate blood culture results due to antibiotic therapy.

34. **(1)** Frontal pain is usually indicative of frontal or ethmoid sinusitis, cerebral tumors, migraine, or problems with the eyes. Occipital or suboccipital pain suggests a cerebellar tumor, occipital neuralgia, sphenoid sinusitis, or tension. Temporal pain can be indicative of tension or lesions in the temporal area of the brain.

35. **(3)** Cerebral vascular disease is not usually included in the differential diagnosis of seizures in a pediatric client. In addition to Options #1, #2, and #4, infection, trauma, tumors, perinatal hypoxia, hypoglycemia, hypocalcemia, vitamin $B_6$ deficiency, phenylketonuria, and drug withdrawal are possible etiologies for a seizure.

36. **(4)** Characteristics of headaches that particularly suggest increased intracranial pressure are headaches that waken the patient from sleep or occur in the morning and that are accompanied by vomiting free of nausea; those related to change of position from prone to supine and from either of those to the erect position; and those related to physical activity (i.e., coughing, sneezing, and straining).

# Pharmacology

37. **(2)** Although most medication is discontinued after 4 years of no seizure activity, this should be confirmed by an EEG. Not all seizure clients require medication; referral to and monitoring by a neurologist are appropriate.

38. **(2)** Hyperplasia of the gums is a common side effect of phenytoin (Dilantin). The child should have regular dental prophylactic hygiene to deal with the problem.

39. **(3)** Infantile spasms are resistant to treatment with most anticonvulsants. The treatment most commonly used is ACTH, administered in a single daily intramuscular dose of 20–40 IU. The benzodiazepines are also effective in controlling infantile spasms. Nitrazepam seems to be more effective than clonazepam (Klonopin) or diazepam (Valium). Valproic acid (Depakene) also is effective therapy for infantile spasms in some infants.

40. **(1)** Occasionally, paradoxical CNS hyperactivity or nervousness may occur. Gingival hyperplasia is associated with phenytoin (Dilantin) use.

# 12

## Gastrointestinal & Liver

## Physical Examination & Diagnostic Tests

1. The nurse practitioner is preparing to examine the abdomen of a child. What is the correct sequence to conduct the examination?

   1. Inspection, palpation, percussion, auscultation.

   2. Palpation, percussion, auscultation, inspection.

   3. Percussion, palpation, auscultation, inspection.

   4. Inspection, auscultation, percussion, palpation.

2. To test for a positive obturator sign in a child with abdominal pain, the nurse practitioner:

   1. Passively rotates the right hip from the 90-degree hip/knee flexion position.

   2. Asks the child to take a deep breath while applying pressure in the area of the gallbladder.

   3. Percusses over the costovertebral angles.

   4. Positions the supine child with hips flexed and auscultates for bowel sounds, then palpates the abdomen, beginning with superficial palpation of nontender areas.

3. Serologic features* of acute hepatitis B are:

   1. HbsAg, HbeAg, and a high titer of IgM anti-HBc.

   2. HbeAg and HbsAg positive.

   3. HbeAg and HbsAg negative.

   4. IgM anti-HBc (high titer) and HbsAg negative.

---

*HBsAg, hepatitis B surface antigen; HBeAg, hepatitis B e antigen; IgM, immunoglobulin M; anti-HBc, antibody to hepatitis B core antigen; anti-HBs, antibody to hepatitis B surface antigen.

4. An older child complains of extreme pain in his abdomen and points to the right lower quadrant. In examining the acute abdomen, the nurse practitioner would:

   1. Immediately order a white blood cell (WBC) count and abdominal x-ray.

   2. Percuss the abdomen in all quadrants, followed by auscultation and gentle palpation.

   3. Palpate the right side of the abdomen first, paying close attention for guarding in the area of pain.

   4. Palpate the left side of the abdomen, then gently palpate the right side, noting guarding and tenderness.

## Disorders

5. Diarrhea is often associated with:

   1. Infectious gastroenteritis, inflammatory bowel disease, diverticulitis.

   2. Diseases of the colon or rectum.

   3. Fever and abdominal pain in sexually transmitted diseases.

   4. Dysuria and flank pain in urinary tract infections.

6. The most important goal of assessing a child with abdominal pain is to:

   1. Palpate the area of pain right away.

   2. Rule out emergent conditions.

   3. Determine the exact etiology of the pain on the first visit for every child.

   4. Determine what tests to order.

7. Which symptoms would the nurse practitioner identify as characteristic of colic?

   1. Diarrhea and abdominal distention.

   2. Unconsolable crying, appropriate weight gain.

   3. Occurs most often in infants 4–6 months old.

   4. Effortless regurgitation and weight loss.

8. Which of the following suggests an emergent condition?

   1. Pain in an adolescent that is rated as 5 on a scale of 1–10 and is relieved by having a bowel movement.

   2. Pain that is progressive, localized, and steady for more than 6 hours and is accompanied by rebound tenderness and guarding.

   3. Pain in an adolescent girl that is sudden in onset, localized in the lower right or left quadrant, and lasts 14–36 hours.

   4. Pain that follows the onset of vomiting and diarrhea.

9. A careful history of an adolescent with a chief complaint of diarrhea reveals that this adolescent has recurrent abdominal pain and diarrhea that alternates with constipation. The most likely diagnosis is:

   1. Drug-induced diarrhea.

   2. Inflammatory bowel disease.

   3. Giardiasis.

   4. Irritable bowel syndrome.

10. Inflammatory toxigenic gastrointestinal illness is characterized by:

    1. Fecal leukocytes, dysentery; site: proximal small bowel.

    2. No fecal leukocytes, watery diarrhea; site: distal small bowel.

    3. Fecal leukocytes, secretory diarrhea; site: colon.

    4. Fecal leukocytes, watery diarrhea; site: colon.

11. Clinical features of irritable bowel syndrome (IBS) include which of the following?

    1. Increased incidence in adolescents.

    2. Affects young children more often than older children.

    3. Increased incidence in males.

    4. No evidence of anxiety and depression in affected children.

12. The nurse practitioner understands that hepatitis B can be transmitted in blood and blood products. Another common mode of transmission of hepatitis B is:

    1. Respiratory contact.

    2. Contaminated fluid.

    3. Fecal–oral route.

    4. Perinatal exposure.

13. An indirect inguinal hernia:

    _Direct_

    1. Is a portion of the bowel or omentum that protrudes directly through the floor of the inguinal canal and exits through the external inguinal ring.

    2. Rarely incarcerates or strangulates.

    3. Is due to a weakness in the abdominal structure.

    4. Passes through the internal abdominal ring, traverses the spermatic cord through the inguinal canal, and exits at the external inguinal ring.

14. Which is true about enterobiasis? _pm worm_

    1. The parasite is in the soil and enters the body through the feet. It can cause anemia. _Hookworm_

    2. The parasite causes pruritus around the anus because the gravid females exit through the anus at night and lay eggs on the skin. The human is the only host of this parasite.

    3. The eggs of this parasite enter the body by ingestion of dirt (pica) or dirt on unwashed vegetables that contain the eggs, or through water containing eggs. _Roundworm_

    4. This parasite is a protozoan. The source is usually contaminated water, but it is spread from person to person by oral–fecal contamination. _giardia_

15. An acute febrile illness with jaundice, anorexia, and malaise; an incubation period of 45–160 days; having a chronic and an acute form; and transmitted by parenteral, sexual, and perinatal routes describes:

    1. Hepatitis A.

    2. Hepatitis B.

    3. Hepatitis C.

    4. Hepatitis D.

16. An adolescent female presents to the nurse practitioner for evaluation of 2 days of increasing crampy, abdominal pain. She states that she also has some mild nausea, anorexia, and a low-grade fever. The client states that the pain is periumbilical. Her STAT complete blood count (CBC) reveals a slightly elevated white count but is otherwise normal. The nurse practitioner's next step for the care of this client is:

    1. Referral to a gynecologist for evaluation of a possible ectopic pregnancy.

    2. Referral to surgeon for evaluation of possible appendicitis.

    3. Observe the client overnight and reassess the next day.

    4. Place the client on a clear liquid diet and have her watch for increasing symptoms.

17. The nurse is interpreting the notation of "string sign" on an upper gastrointestinal tract series performed on an infant. This is associated with a diagnosis of:

    1. Intussusception.

    2. Aganglionic congenital megacolon.

    3. Pyloric stenosis.

    4. Esophageal atresia.

18. The nurse practitioner identifies which of these conditions as most conducive to the development of metabolic alkalosis in a child?

    1. Severe anxiety resulting in hyperventilation.

    2. Excessive vomiting related to gastroenteritis.

    3. Depressed respirations from excessive narcotics ingestion.

    4. Decreased renal function with glomeruli damage.

19. The nurse practitioner in the emergency room examines a child who has severe diarrhea and vomiting resulting in dehydration. One of the orders is to start an IV of 500 ml normal saline with 10 mEq of potassium to run at 23 ml/hr. The child is NPO. What would be a priority action prior to initiating the IV fluid?

    1. Weigh the child.
    2. Obtain serum electrolyte values.
    3. Make sure the child is voiding adequately.
    4. Determine amount of previous fluid loss.

20. A young child is brought to the clinic by her mother complaining of abrupt onset of vomiting followed by over 10 liquid stools with mucus for the past 48 hours. The temperature is 100°F orally. The stool smear by the nurse practitioner is negative for WBCs. The most likely etiologic pathogen for this young child's gastroenteritis is:

    1. Rotavirus.
    2. *Shigella dysenteriae.*
    3. *Camphylobacter jejuni.*
    4. *Salmonella.*

21. The symptoms of abdominal discomfort associated with meals, diarrhea or constipation, anorexia, weight loss, failure to grow, and failure to develop sexually are most associated with:

    1. Ulcerative colitis.
    2. Irritable bowel syndrome.
    3. Hirschsprung's disease.
    4. Crohn's disease.

22. What question by the nurse practitioner would be appropriate to ask the parents of an infant who is suspected of having intussusception?

    1. "Does the infant have clay-colored stools?"
    2. "Does the infant have projectile vomiting?"
    3. "Does the infant have constant abdominal pain?"

    4. "Does the infant have red currant jelly stools?"

23. The major symptom of reflux in infants is:

    1. Vomiting or regurgitation, especially after feeding.
    2. Poor weight gain.
    3. Hyperirritability and refusal of feeding.
    4. Fever and diarrhea.

24. Medical therapy for young infants with vomiting or regurgitation of gastroesophageal reflux disease (GERD) consists of the following:

    1. Small feedings and burping after each feeding.
    2. Placing the infant prone after feedings.
    3. Placing the infant supine in the infant seat after feedings.
    4. Thicken the feedings.

25. A baby is born to a mother who is HBsAg positive. Which is true regarding the management of the baby?

    1. No prophylaxis against hepatitis B needs to be given to the baby.
    2. This baby should have one dose of hepatitis B immune globulin administered.
    3. This baby should have one dose of hepatitis B vaccine administered by the nurse practitioner.
    4. This baby should have one dose of hepatitis B immune globulin and a complete three-dose immunization of hepatitis B vaccine.

26. What physical findings would lead the nurse practitioner to suspect Hirschsprung's disease in a 6-month-old infant?

    1. Rectal bleeding, diarrhea, and prolonged jaundice at birth.
    2. History of constipation and current abdominal distention.
    3. Irritability, vomiting, and dehydration.
    4. History of colic, bloody diarrhea, and nausea.

27. A common cause of acute abdominal pain in children <5 years old is:

    1. Appendicitis.

    2. Intussusception.

    3. Incarcerated hernia.

    4. Gastroenteritis.

28. The nurse practitioner understands that common causes of recurrent abdominal pain in adolescents are:

    1. Intussusception, gastroenteritis, peptic ulcer disease, and right lower lobe pneumonia.

    2. Psychogenic pain, mittelschmerz, trauma, and urinary tract infections.

    3. Parasitic infestation, musculoskeletal pain, dysmenorrhea, and chronic stool retention.

    4. Incarcerated hernia, appendicitis, inflammatory bowel disease.

29. An adolescent client is brought to the nurse practitioner by his mother for evaluation after a dirt bike accident. The client states that the bike flipped over and struck him on the abdomen. There is a hematoma noted just below the left anterior rib area. In this case, the nurse practitioner must be particularly aware of the possibility of:

    1. Ruptured bowel due to blunt trauma.

    2. Bladder trauma.

    3. Hypovolemia due to ruptured spleen.

    4. Dysrhythmias.

30. A 2-year-old Asian-American child comes to the clinic with her parents and infant brother. The chief complaint is abdominal pain and flatulence and diarrhea after eating. Until 3 months ago, she had continued to be breast-fed twice a day. The nurse practitioner would suspect:

    1. Irritable bowel syndrome.

    2. Hirschsprung's disease.

    3. Lactose intolerance.

    4. Food allergy.

31. A 10-year-old girl comes to the clinic with complaints of nausea, vomiting, and right upper quadrant pain during vigorous play. She is also more tired than usual. Serologic test for IgM antibodies are ordered to rule out:

    1. Cholecystitis.

    2. Hepatitis A.

    3. Infectious mononucleosis.

    4. Hepatitis B.

32. A 3-year-old presents to the clinic with diffuse abdominal pain, irritability, and a low-grade fever. The mother states the toddler has not had a bowel movement since the previous morning. Physical exam reveals umbilical tenderness, guarding, and hypoactive bowel sounds. The nurse practitioner's next step is to:

    1. Refer to a physician/surgeon for further evaluation.

    2. Assess for rebound tenderness and do a rectal exam.

    3. Prescribe a pediatric Fleets enema.

    4. Assess dietary intake for past 24 hours.

33. A 2-year-old child is seen for a foreign body in the gastrointestinal tract. The nurse practitioner pays particular attention to the size of the object, knowing that passing the ligament of Treitz is difficult with objects larger than:

    1. 5 cm.    *thin muscle connecting the junction*
    *≑ the duodenum & jejunum*
    2. 8 cm.    *marked the 1st end, 2nd*
    *begining of bowel*
    3. 10 cm.

    4. 12 cm.

34. A 2-month-old infant presents with coughing that results in emesis, which occurs when laid supine after eating. The infant has lost 1.3 lb since birth, with a birth weight of 7.5 lb. The nurse practitioner focuses her assessment toward the possibility of:

    1. Suck–swallow incoordination.

    2. Gastroesophageal reflux.

    3. Tracheoesophageal fistula.

    4. Infantile colic.

35. A child has been diagnosed with bacterial gastroenteritis. *Campylobacter jejuni* has been cultured. The nurse practitioner understands that *Campylobacter* gastroenteritis:

    1. Begins with watery diarrhea, high fever, and malaise followed 24 hours later by tenesmus and frank dysentery; children rarely need oral hydration therapy.

    2. Is associated with recurrent abdominal pain (RAP syndrome) and needs to have three repeat stool cultures to confirm diagnosis.

    3. Is responsible for more than 50% of the cases of acute diarrhea in children (*Campylobacter* is the most common infectious agent in infants).

    4. Begins with fever and malaise, followed by nausea, vomiting, profuse bloody diarrhea, and abdominal pain.

36. A 16-year-old female client presents to the emergency room and is seen by the nurse practitioner. The client had a gradual onset of abdominal pain, starting in the periumbilical region and now in the right lower quadrant. It is accompanied by nausea, anorexia, constipation, and low-grade fever. The physical exam confirms the diagnosis of acute appendicitis. What diagnostic studies are **least** useful in confirming this diagnosis?

    1. CBC with differential.

    2. Flat plate of abdomen and of kidney, ureter, and bladder (KUB).

    3. Pelvic ultrasound.

    4. Pregnancy test.

## Pharmacology

37. After percutaneous or perimucosal exposure to a HBsAg-positive source:

    1. In an unvaccinated person, begin the hepatitis B series.

    2. In a known hepatitis B responder with an adequate response, no treatment is necessary.

    3. In known hepatitis B responder with inadequate anti-HBs, give hepatitis B immune globulin (HBIG) and initiate a new hepatitis B vaccine series.

    4. In an unknown hepatitis B responder who competed the entire hepatitis B vaccine series, give a hepatitis B booster.

38. After exposure to household or sexual contacts with hepatitis A, the nurse practitioner would:

    1. Give immunoglobulin 0.02 ml/kg as soon as possible but no later than 2 weeks after exposure.

    2. Give HBIG × 1 and immunoglobulin 0.02 ml/kg as soon as possible.

    3. Give immunoglobulin 0.02 ml/kg and HBIG × 2.

    4. Understand that no injections are needed.

39. Shigellosis is treated by:

    1. No medication intervention, careful toileting and bathroom sanitation, and keeping the perineal area clean.

    2. Symptomatic treatment and antidiarrheal agents.

    3. Symptomatic treatment and trimethoprim-sulfamethoxazole (Septra) dosed for age and weight bid × 5 days.

    4. Boiling water and quinacrine HCI (Atabrine) 100 mg PO tid × 5 days.

40. Pharmacologic management of nausea and vomiting in children includes:

    1. Benzquinamide (Emete-Con) .5–1 mg q 3–4 hours IM.

    2. Promethazine (Phenergan) 25 mg suppository for children over 6 years.

    3. Hydroxyzine hydrochloride (Vistaril) 1 mg IM for children over 12 years.

    4. Trimethobenzamide (Tigan) 10 mg PO for children over 12 years.

41. An adolescent presents with a history of recent unprotected sexual activity with a partner now diagnosed with hepatitis B. She is currently asymptomatic and she does

not recall having a vaccine in the past. The best action for the nurse practitioner is:

1. Draw a anti-HBe test.

2. Administer one dose of HBIG.

3. Administer two doses of HBIG and initiate vaccination.

4. Administer one dose of HBIG and initiate vaccination.

42. A 3-year-old child is seen in the clinic for chronic, relapsing diarrhea. A stool for ova and parasites is obtained and is positive for *Giardia*. The most appropriate pharmacologic intervention would be:

1. Ampicillin (Omnipen).

2. Erythromycin (E-Mycin).

3. Metronidazole (Flagyl).

4. Tetracycline (Achromycin).

43. An 8-year-old child has retentive encopresis. Pharmacologic management includes:

1. Hyperphosphate enemas (two or three) to remove impaction and mineral oil.

2. Dicyclomine (Bentyl) 10 mg tid PO qd.

3. Phenolphthalein (Ex-Lax) prn to prevent constipation.

4. Imipramine (Tofranil) 25 mg PO qd initially, increase to 50 mg in 1 week.

Tenesmus: cramping, rectal pain. A distressing but ineffectual urge to evacuate the rectum or bladder

Shigellosis — Bactrim
giardiasis — Flagyl

# 12  Answers & Rationales

## Physical Examination & Diagnostic Tests

1. **(4)** Inspection and auscultation should be conducted first in order to prevent undue guarding. If the examination is painful initially, the client is going to be very uncomfortable with allowing the examiner to continue.

2. **(1)** If abdominal pain results from passive internal rotation of the right hip from the 90-degree hip/knee flexion position, the child has a positive obturator sign, which is suggestive of appendicitis. In a positive Murphy's sign (Option #2), pain and a brief inspiratory arrest result when a child takes a deep breath while the examiner applies pressure over the gallbladder. This is suggestive of cholecystitis. Percussion over the costovertebral angles that elicits pain is a positive costovertebral angle tenderness suggestive of pyelonephritis. Positioning of the client in a supine position with hips flexed and then auscultating and palpating the abdomen, beginning with light palpation in nontender areas, is the sequence for examining the abdomen.

3. **(1)** HbsAg is found in active or chronic hepatitis B disease. HbeAg indicates active replication of the virus. IgM anti-Hbs indicates chronic disease. Positive HbsAg indicates chronic disease, and negative HbsAg indicates prior exposure.

4. **(4)** Always palpate the nontender areas first, before going to the area of pain and tenderness. Option #2 does not describe the correct order of assessing an abdomen,

which is inspection, auscultation, percussion, and palpation. Although Option #1 may be done, it does not answer what the question is asking.

## Disorders

5. **(1)** Diarrhea is a common symptom in infectious gastroenteritis, inflammatory bowel disease, diverticulitis, and early intestinal obstruction. Diseases of the colon or rectum are often associated with constipation that clearly precedes the onset of abdominal pain. With sexually transmitted diseases, abdominal pain can often occur with vaginal discharge or bleeding and sometimes irregular menses. Dysuria, flank pain, hematuria, and urinary frequency are common signs and symptoms of upper or lower urinary tract infections or ureteral calculi.

6. **(2)** The most important goal in evaluating a child who presents with abdominal pain is to rule out emergent conditions. Palpation is done after auscultation. Begin in an area away from the site of the pain. It is important to rule out emergent causes and ideal to make an exact diagnosis every time. However, due to the sometimes complicated nature of abdominal pain, it is not always possible to do this. Ordering appropriate laboratory tests is important but is not the most important goal.

7. **(2)** Colic is defined as paroxysmal infant crying which increases through the 4th to 6th week and often disappears by 3–4 months.

8. **(2)** Localized pain that steadily increases for 6 or more hours with rebound tenderness and guarding could be caused by an emergent condition, such as appendicitis or ruptured ectopic pregnancy. Pain in an adolescent girl that is relieved by having a bowel movement could be constipation; pain that is sudden in onset and is in the right lower quadrant, lasting 14–36 hours could be mittelschmerz, if the girl is midway through her menstrual cycle. Pain that follows the onset of vomiting and diarrhea usually occurs in gastroenteritis.

9. **(4)** Irritable bowel syndrome presents with abdominal pain and/or altered bowel habits. These symptoms can be aggravated by psychological stresses. Symptoms disappear while sleeping. Bacterial or viral gastroenteritis presents as abdominal pain with diarrhea and vomiting of abrupt onset. Drug-induced diarrhea follows initiation of drug therapy, and in this situation there is no mention of previous drug therapy. In inflammatory bowel disease, nocturnal diarrhea and abdominal pain are often accompanied by rectal fistula, fever, and/or skin lesions. Diarrhea occurring with giardiasis is malodorous. Weight loss occurs over a period of weeks.

10. **(3)** The etiologic agents that produce inflammation and cause diarrhea are characterized by positive fecal leukocytes. Viral diarrhea is free of pus, thus no fecal leukocytes would be found on the smear. Noninflammatory diarrhea is usually caused by rotavirus. Toxigenic bacteria cause diarrhea by elaborating toxins that have been released after bacterial growth in the intestines. These poisonous substances result in secretory diarrhea.

11. **(1)** There is no evidence of increased incidence in males or females in pediatric clients. There is increased anxiety and depression in affected children. Psychogenic factors are not thought to cause IBS, but these factors do influence the progress.

12. **(4)** A common means of hepatitis B transmission is from mother to baby, perinatally. Other mechanisms of transmission are by infected body fluids, sexual contact, and parenterally. Hepatitis E virus is spread in contaminated water. Hepatitis A's mode of transmission is fecal–oral and person-to-person.

13. **(4)** Because indirect hernias are due to a congenital defect in which the processus vaginalis remains patent, they occur more often in younger persons. A portion of the bowel and/or the omentum comes through the internal abdominal ring, traverses the spermatic cord through the inguinal canal, and exits at the external inguinal ring. In a direct hernia, the omentum or bowel protrudes directly through the floor of the inguinal canal and exits through the external inguinal ring.

14. **(2)** These parasites reside in the intestine. Females lay eggs on the skin outside the anus, resulting in extreme pruritus. The only host is humans. Hookworm larvae reside in the soil, enter the body through the feet, and can cause anemia. When dirt containing roundworm eggs is ingested due to pica or on unwashed vegetables or contaminated water is consumed, an intestinal infestation occurs. Giardiasis results from ingestion of the protozoan *Giardia lamblia* through contaminated water or via oral–fecal transmission.

15. **(2)** These characteristics describe hepatitis B. Hepatitis A has similar symptoms but can be transmitted by the oral–fecal or oral–genital route and has an incubation period of 15–50 days and no chronic form. Hepatitis C infection rarely causes jaundice. It is transmitted parenterally and has an incubation period of 14–140 days and a chronic form. Hepatitis D coexists with hepatitis B, is transmitted parenterally, and can also become chronic. Hepatitis E is characterized by oral–fecal transmission associated with contaminated food and water, an incubation period of 14–60 days, and no chronic disease state.

16. **(2)** Increasing crampy abdominal pain that starts as periumbilical pain, anorexia, and fever are classic symptoms of appendicitis. The client should be evaluated by a surgeon to decease the risk of rupture of the appendix. While ectopic pregnancy should always be a consideration in young females with abdominal pain, the characteristics of the pain and other symptoms are not typical of an ectopic pregnancy.

17. **(3)** The string sign is indicative of a narrow pyloric channel and is associated with pyloric stenosis. Intussusception would be evaluated by a barium enema. Hirschsprung's disease can be diagnosed by doing a Wagenstein-Rice series (air rises in the inflated colon).

18. **(2)** Excessive vomiting with loss of acid is a common problem with metabolic alkalosis. Respiratory problems do not precipitate primary metabolic acid–base imbalance, and renal disease most often causes metabolic acidosis.

19. **(3)** It is critical that a child be voiding prior to starting an IV solution with potassium. Renal compromise is always a possibility, and adequate output should be established prior to initiating fluid.

20. **(1)** Rotavirus is the most frequent cause of gastroenteritis in children ages 6 months to 2 years. The Norwalk virus is more predominant in school-age children. Up to 58% of diarrhea in children is due to viral causes. Viral causes result in vomiting and then diarrhea. The stool smear is negative for WBCs in viral causes and positive in bacterial causes (Options #2, #3, and #4). In viral diarrhea, the fever is mild and the diarrhea is watery and nonbloody.

21. **(4)** Crohn's clinical features include severe weight loss, abdominal pain, growth failure, and weight loss. In irritable bowel syndrome abdominal pain predominates. Altered bowel habits with either diarrhea or constipation are also seen. Hirschsprung's disease is characterized by progressive abdominal distention and lack of passage of a normal bowel movement. Ulcerative colitis clinical features include diarrhea, rectal bleeding, and moderate weight loss.

22. **(4)** Red currant jelly stools are seen in intussusception and are caused by a mixture of stool, mucus, and blood. Clay-colored stools are seen with hepatitis. Projectile vomiting is associated with pyloric stenosis. Infants with intussusception usually have periods of severe pain followed by intervals in which they appear comfortable.

23. **(1)** The major symptom of reflux is vomiting or regurgitation. It may occur in sleep and frequently after feeding. Poor weight gain, hyperirritability, and refusal of feeding may be signs in some infants but are not the major symptom. Fever or diarrhea may be present in clients with acute otitis media, gastroenteritis, or urinary tract infections.

24. **(1)** The optimal therapy for GERD should include frequent small feedings, burping after each feeding, and placing the baby prone on a surface inclined at 30 degrees. The flat prone position is not advocated as it allows gravity to promote reflux. The supine position leads to more reflux as compared with prone. Proof of the effectiveness of thickening feedings has not been demonstrated.

25. **(4)** For an infant born to a HBsAg-positive mother, the recommendations are one dose of hepatitis B immune globulin (by 12 hours after birth) and a complete three-dose immunization of hepatitis B vaccine. The vaccine will stimulate the newborn's active immunity.

26. **(2)** Classic signs and symptoms of Hirschsprung's disease in later infancy include alternating diarrhea and constipation and abdominal distention. The stools are offensive and ribbon-like, the abdomen is enlarged, and the veins are prominent.

27. **(4)** Gastroenteritis is the most common cause of abdominal pain in all age groups. The incidence of appendicitis increases after the age of 5. Intussusception and incarcerated hernias are not common events and certainly occur less often than gastroenteritis.

28. **(3)** Parasitic infestations cause recurrent episodes of abdominal pain, often with diarrhea, nausea, and vomiting, depending on the type of infestation. Musculoskeletal pain is usually sharp and recurs with various activities or body movements that trigger the pain. Dysmenorrhea accompanies or precedes menses. Chronic stool retention occurs in a child with a history of ineffective toilet training. There is often a family history of constipation. All of the other conditions present with an acute symptoms, except for psychogenic pain, which is recurrent and is a diagnosis of exclusion, and mittelschmerz, which may occur monthly.

29. **(3)** The location of the injury indicates the possibility of a ruptured spleen. While bowel and bladder problems are possible with blunt trauma to the abdomen, the upper abdominal location makes a spleen injury more likely.

30. **(3)** Lactose intolerance is common among Asian clients. The primary symptoms are bloating, flatulence, abdominal cramps, and diarrhea to 2 hours after lactose-containing food consumption.

31. **(2)** Right upper quadrant pain during exercise along with malaise, nausea, and vomiting are early signs of hepatitis A. Elevated IgM antibodies indicate a recent/current infection.

32. **(2)** Further physical examination is needed to rule out appendicitis (although rare, it can occur in young children). Further diagnostic testing and assessment would also be needed for differential diagnosis of lactose intolerance, urinary tract infection, or extra-abdominal causes.

33. **(1)** Objects 3–4 cm or larger have difficulty passing the ligament of Treitz and other points of narrowing, such as the cardioesophageal junction.

34. **(2)** Increased abdominal pressure with the infant in a supine position after eating can result in passage of gastric contents into the esophagus; during sleep the gastric contents can frequently be aspirated, resulting in the forceful coughing and resultant emesis. Suck–swallow incoordination can cause the same problems regardless of position, as will a tracheoesophageal fistula.

35. **(4)** These accurately describe the symptoms of *Campylobacter* gastroenteritis. Option #1 describes *Shigella* gastroenteritis; however, dehydration is common with *Shigella* and oral rehydration is often necessary. Option #2 is an incorrect statement. Option #3 describes rotavirus.

36. **(3)** The pelvic ultrasound is not a useful test to obtain for appendicitis as it will not allow for adequate examination of the appendix. The CBC with differential is useful due to the expected rise in WBC count seen in this inflammatory state. The flat plate of the abdomen and KUB are very helpful to determine the extent of the problem and rule out other diagnoses. Since pregnancy can cause these symptoms if ectopic, the nurse practitioner should consider it as part of the differential diagnosis.

## Pharmacology

37. **(2)** If a person exposed to a client known to be positive for hepatitis B has sufficient immunity to hepatitis B, no treatment is necessary. If this same person had not been vaccinated, in addition to initiation of the hepatitis B vaccine series, HBIG 0.06 ml/kg IM is also administered. If an exposed person has had an inadequate immune response to the hepatitis B vaccine series, a hepatitis B booster is to be given. There is no need to repeat the series. If the response to the hepatitis B vaccine series is unknown, test the exposed person's hepatitis D surface antigen level and decide what intervention, if any, is needed.

38. **(1)** To minimize the risk of a contact developing hepatitis A, immunoglobulin 0.02 ml/kg should be given as soon as possible after exposure. It has not been shown to be effective if administered more than 2 weeks after exposure.

39. **(3)** Treatment with trimethoprim-sulfamethoxazole shortens the course and prevents further spread of the organism. Prevention of dehydration that can result from the diarrhea is accomplished through symptomatic treatment (clear liquids for 24–48 hours, no dairy products, electrolyte-rich sports drinks, advance diet as tolerated). Antidiarrheal medications are not recommended because intestinal motility is important in recovery. Option #4 would be appropriate treatment for nonpregnant adults who have giardiasis.

40. **(2)** The recommended antiemetic, if one must be used is Phenergan, and it should not be given to children under 2 years. Emete-Con is not given to children. Tigan is dosed at 100–200 mg, not 10 mg. The dosage for Vistaril is 25–100 mg, and it is not recommended for control of vomiting in children.

41. **(4)** For unvaccinated adolescents with exposure to hepatitis B, administer one dose of HBIG and initiate the vaccine. If clients think they may have been vaccinated, but they do not know if they responded, the nurse practitioner may have a prevaccination antibody testing done. The anti-HBe test is done to determine the potential for transmission; it generally appears about 3 months after the onset of the infection.

42. **(3)** The drug of choice for treating *Giardia* is metronidazole 5 mg/kg (up to 250 mg) tid × 5 days (80–90% effective). This drug is well tolerated in children. Metronidazole does have a disulfiram-like effect and should not be used in children or adolescents receiving ethanol-containing medications. All of the other drugs are ineffective for *Giardia*. Tetracycline should never be prescribed to children under age 8 for any reason.

43. **(1)** Hyperphosphate enemas (two or three) to remove impaction and mineral oil 15 ml/10 kg to keep the stools soft is the recommended pharmacologic management, along with a nonconstipating high-fiber diet and sitting on the toilet for at least 10 minutes tid. Bentyl is indicated for irritable bowel syndrome. Ex-Lax is a stimulant laxative and is not recommended for children. Tofranil is indicated for enuresis.

# 13

# Hematology

## Physical Examination & Diagnostic Tests

1. The nurse practitioner describes a "shotty" lymph node as:

   1. Tender, mobile, and >5 mm.
   2. Small and pellet-like.
   3. Discrete and cystic.
   4. Irregular, soft, and fixed to surrounding tissue.

2. In examining lymph nodes, the nurse practitioner understands:

   1. Children are more likely to develop generalized lymphadenopathy than adults in response to a mild infection.
   2. Adolescents frequently have enlarged, nontender supraclavicular and epitrochlear lymph nodes due to growing.
   3. Lymphadenopathy in an adolescent indicates acute or chronic infection and rarely malignancy.
   4. Enlarged neck lymph nodes in children with no other physical findings are highly suspicious of Burkitt's lymphoma.

3. The most sensitive test for the diagnosis of sickle cell anemia is:

   1. Complete blood count (CBC) with a peripheral smear.
   2. Bone marrow biopsy and aspiration.
   3. Hemoglobin electrophoresis. to look for Hgb S
   4. Hemoglobin and hematocrit.

4. A school-age child presents to the clinic. His mother reports a recent history of easy fatiguability ("he can't keep up with his brother anymore"), unexplained bruising, and that he has been treated for an upper respiratory infection with multiple antibiotics over the past 6 months. Physical exam reveals scattered bruising in no apparent pattern, pallor, and cervical lymphadenopathy. The diagnostic work-up for this child should include:

   1. Chest x-ray and electrocardiogram.
   2. Liver function tests and an abdominal ultrasound.
   3. Prothrombin time (PT) and partial thromboplastin time (PTT).
   4. CBC with differential and platelet count.

5. In evaluating the laboratory findings on a child with iron deficiency anemia, the nurse practitioner expects:

   1. Mean corpuscular volume (MCV) 80 and reticulocyte count low.

   2. MCV 120 and hemoglobin 12 gm.

   3. MCV 99 and hematocrit 34%.

   4. MCV 96 and normal reticulocyte count.

   *immature RBG*

6. The nurse practitioner explains a bone marrow aspiration procedure to a 4-year-old child. Which behavior of the child would reflect effective teaching?

   1. Appears calm as the nurse takes her for the procedure.

   2. Asks if she can have ice cream after the procedure.

   3. States that her blood is bad and the doctor will make it better.

   4. Points at her doll saying that "They have to put a needle here to look at my blood."

7. What is the anemia screening recommendation according to the American Academy of Pediatrics?

   1. Every other year starting at age 1.

   2. Semiannually.

   3. One time between the age span of 15 months and 4 years.

   4. At the first-month well-child visit.

8. An adolescent female presents to the nurse practitioner's office with complaints of fatigue, dizziness, decreased activity tolerance, and occasional bounding heart rate. Physical examination reveals pallor (including mucous membranes), tachycardia, and general appearance of lethargy. The following tests are ordered: CBC with differential, peripheral smear, serum iron, total iron-binding capacity (TIBC), and serum ferritin. These tests are ordered because there is a high index of suspicion of:

   1. Sideroblastic anemia.

   2. Megaloblastic anemia.

   3. Folic acid deficiency anemia.

   4. Iron deficiency anemia.

9. Anemia of chronic disease would reveal which of the following lab findings?

   1. Decreased iron, decreased TIBC, and decreased serum ferritin.

   2. Decreased iron, decreased TIBC, and increased serum ferritin.

   3. Decreased iron, increased TIBC, and decreased serum ferritin. *Fe def anem>*

   4. Decreased iron, increased TIBC, and increased serum ferritin.

## Disorders

10. Sickle cell anemia is caused by:

    1. Exposure to ionizing radiation.

    2. A genetically induced production of abnormal hemoglobin S.

    3. A deficiency of dietary folic acid.

    4. Long-term use of thiazide diuretics.

11. A young adult client has a folic acid deficiency anemia. The nurse practitioner teaches the client to eat foods rich in folic acid such as:

    1. Green leafy vegetables, nuts, and liver.

    2. Carrots, salmon, and avocados.

    3. Cottage cheese, yogurt, and skim milk.

    4. Lima beans, brussel sprouts, and potatoes.

12. Iron deficiency anemia is an example of:

    1. Macrocytic, normochromic anemia.

    2. Macrocytic, hypochromic anemia.

    *MCV    small    pale*

    3. Microcytic, hypochromic anemia.

    4. Normocytic, normochromic anemia.

13. The nurse practitioner explains to the family of a child diagnosed with acute idiopathic thrombocytopenia purpura (ITP) that:

1. It is generally a long-term problem that has a poor prognosis and does not respond to corticosteroid treatment.

2. Life-threatening hemorrhage and intracranial bleeding occurs in 80% of the cases.

3. It is a result of decreased removal of platelets from the circulation by macrophage cells of the reticuloendothelial system.

4. It is a temporary bleeding disorder with the majority of children recovering completely within one year of diagnosis.

14. Anemia of chronic disease is a:

   1. Normochromic, normocytic anemia.

   2. Normochromic, microcytic anemia.

   3. Hypochromic, microcytic anemia.

   4. Hypochromic, macrocytic anemia.

15. What would be the primary prevention recommendation to prevent iron deficiency anemia in a toddler?

   1. Encourage high-potency, iron-fortified vitamin supplementation starting at birth.

   2. Obtain a screening hemoglobin and hematocrit at ages 1 and 3 years.

   3. Have mother purchase iron-fortified cereal.

   4. Encourage breast-feeding or iron-enriched formula during infancy.

16. A young adult presents to the clinic for a routine checkup. History is unremarkable and, on physical exam, an enlarged (2-cm), mobile, nontender, and rubbery lymph node is palpated on the left posterior cervical chain. The nurse practitioner's next step is:

   1. Order a throat culture and monospot.

   2. Refer to a surgeon for a lymph node biopsy.

   3. Order a STAT chest x-ray.

   4. No intervention is necessary at this time.

17. The nurse practitioner understands that "B" symptoms associated with non-Hodgkin's lymphoma (NHL) include:

   1. Bruising and bleeding.

   2. Peripheral edema, shortness of breath, and ascites.

   3. Fever, night sweats, and unexplained weight loss (>10% of body weight).

   4. Headache, fatigue, and weakness.

18. In teaching the parents of a child with anemia to include foods rich in iron in the diet, the nurse practitioner encourages the preparation of what foods?

   1. Cheese, milk, and yogurt.

   2. Red beans, whole-grain bread, and bran cereal.

   3. Tomatoes, cabbage, and citrus fruits.

   4. Beef, spinach, and peanut butter.

19. The nurse practitioner is concerned about the development of which complication in a young child with a diagnosis of iron deficiency anemia?

   1. Crohn's disease.

   2. Megaloblastic anemia. from ↓ B12 & folic acid

   3. Impaired cognitive development.

   4. Hepatic and spleen dysfunction.

20. The nurse practitioner is counseling a client who has a child with sickle cell disease. The client asks "If my child has sickle cell disease, does that mean that I am at an increased risk for developing the same problems?" The nurse practitioner's response would be based on what principle of sickle cell disease?

   1. The mother is at an increased risk because the condition is inherited; she probably has the condition and has not had an active episode.

   2. There is no risk for the mother developing the condition, as males are the carriers of the trait.

   3. There is a 25% chance that the mother will be affected by the disease, especially at times of stress.

   4. The parents are both carriers of the trait, but they do not have the active disease; each child has a 25% chance of having the condition.

21. During a clinic visit, the nurse practitioner notes that an 11-month-old is pale. The physical examination reveals: pulse 170, height 25th percentile, weight 95th percentile. The nurse practitioner questions the mother about the infant's diet. The mother states that the infant eats mostly pureed fruits and whole milk. The nurse practitioner expects which diagnostic finding?

    1. Normal hemoglobin.

    2. Elevated MCV.

    3. Low serum ferritin level.

    4. Macrocytic, hyperchromic anemia.

22. The nurse practitioner knows that an infant who is exclusively breast-fed is at risk for developing iron deficiency anemia at:

    1. 1 month of age.

    2. 2 months of age.

    3. 4 months of age.

    4. 6 months of age.

23. The anemia associated with plumbism is:

    1. Microcytic, hypochromic.

    2. Macrocytic, hyperchromic.

    3. Normocytic, normochromic.

    4. Normocytic, hyperchromic.

24. All of the following are associated with hemophilia except:

    1. Hemarthrosis.

    2. Henoch-Schönlein purpura.

    3. Superficial hematomas.

    4. Hematuria.

## Pharmacology

25. Treatment of anemia of chronic disease should include:

    1. A folic supplement, 1 mg PO qd.

    2. Iron sulfate ($FeSO_4$) supplement, 300 mg PO tid.

    3. Treatment of the underlying condition.

    4. Weekly epoetin alfa (Epogen) injections.

26. A toddler has been diagnosed as having iron deficiency anemia and the nurse practitioner has prescribed elemental iron 6 mg/kg/day in three divided doses. Instructions to give the parents would include:

    1. Give the iron with food to increase the absorption of the medication.

    2. Give the medication through a straw to decrease the staining of the teeth.

    3. Avoid foods containing ascorbic acid because it will decrease the absorption of the medication.

    4. If a dose is missed, double up on the next two doses.

27. Important teaching for a family who has a child with hemophilia that needs to be taught to administer antihemophilic factor (AHF) is:

    1. After medication is reconstituted, it is stable for a week at room temperature.

    2. Discard reconstituted medication if it is clear and slightly yellow in color.

    3. Do not refrigerate or freeze reconstituted AHF.

    4. To dissolve, vigorously shake to promote rapid dissolution.

# 13   Answers & Rationales

## Physical Examination & Diagnostic Tests

1. **(2)** Shotty, or small and pellet-like, lymph nodes that are movable, cool, nontender, discrete, and up to 3 mm in diameter are usually considered normal.

2. **(1)** Children often have generalized lymphadenopathy in response to mild infections of the skin or respiratory tract. Palpable lymph nodes are generally not present in healthy individuals; however, some individuals may have small, discrete, nontender nodes that are not clinically significant. Enlarged lymph nodes may indicate infection, inflammation, and malignancy in both child and adult. A painless, firm supraclavicular or cervical lymph node is a common sign for Hodgkin's disease in children, not Burkitt's lymphoma, with which the child has other associated symptoms depending on the system affected.

3. **(3)** Normal and abnormal hemoglobins can be detected by electrophoresis, which matches hemolyzed red cell material against standard bands for the various known hemoglobins, including hemoglobin S (the abnormal hemoglobin that is associated with sickle cell anemia). CBC with peripheral smear and hemoglobin/hematocrit would not yield enough information to diagnose sickle cell anemia. Bone marrow biopsy would not be necessary and would not indicate the presence of hemoglobin S.

4. **(4)** This clinical presentation would make the practitioner consider the diagnosis of leukemia, necessitating a work-up. A CBC with differential, along with platelet count (indicators of bone marrow function), is diagnostic for leukemia. Further testing may be necessary, but the work-up should always include a CBC.

5. **(1)** The findings associated with iron deficiency anemia include a low MCV (<90), decreased hemoglobin and hematocrit, and a low reticulocyte count. An elevated MCV is associated with macrocytic anemias (i.e., pernicious anemia).

6. **(4)** Dolls and puppets are effective teaching tools for the preschool child. Using the doll reflects the child's understanding of the procedure. Children will often withdraw and appear calm when they have feelings of anxiety.

7. **(3)** The peak age for iron deficiency anemia is at 18 months. Remember to look for a range (i.e., a beginning and ending date for recommendations).

8. **(4)** This client's clinical picture is a classic presentation for anemia. Further testing would be needed to determine the type of anemia involved. The most common cause in adolescent girls would be due to poor nutritional intake and having menses. Megalobastic anemia is due to deficient intake of vitamin $B_{12}$ and/or folic acid. The tests that were ordered would confirm or rule out this diagnosis; the peripheral smear is especially important in diagnosing the specific type of anemia. If the smear ruled out the diagnosis of iron deficiency anemia, it would lead the practitioner to other diagnoses (including the remaining choices) and appropriate laboratory tests required for confirmation.

9. **(2)** Normal to increased iron stores (serum ferritin) with concurrent low serum iron is the hallmark finding of anemia of chronic disease. The serum iron is decreased along with the total iron binding capacity. Options #1 and #4 contain incorrect information for the anemias. Option #3 contains the findings for iron deficiency anemia.

## Disorders

10. **(2)** Sickle cell anemia is a genetic disorder characterized by the production of hemoglobin S, an anemia secondary to shortened erythrocyte survival, microvascular occlusion by sickle-shaped erythrocytes, and an increased susceptibility to certain infections. Exposure to ionizing radiation has been associated with the development of certain malignancies, especially leukemia. A deficiency of dietary folic acid does not cause sickle cell anemia, although folic acid is used in the treatment of these clients to help increase hematopoiesis and aid in recovery from aplastic events. Long-term use of thiazide diuretics has been implicated in the development of hemolytic or aplastic anemias, in very rare cases.

11. **(1)** Green leafy vegetables, nuts, and liver are excellent sources of folic acid. Also, cereals and breads are now fortified with folic acid. The other foods are not significant sources of folic acid.

12. **(3)** Iron deficiency anemia is a microcytic, hypochromic anemia. The red blood cells are smaller (microcytic) due to the decrease in hemoglobin production caused by inadequate amounts of iron. This also makes the cell appear pale (hypochromic). The other selections describe other types of anemia, and would be determined by the peripheral smear.

13. **(1)** Acute idiopathic thrombocytopenia purpura (ITP) is a temporary bleeding disorder characterized by severe thrombocytopenia and bleeding (treated with corticosteroids or high doses of IV immunoglobulin) with the majority of children recovering completely within one year of diagnosis. Less than 1% of children have an experience with life-threatening hemorrhage or intracranial bleeding. The pathophysiology is due to an *increased* removal of platelets from the circulation by macrophage cells of the reticuloendothelial system.

14. **(1)** Anemia of chronic disease is a chronic normochromic, normocytic anemia. There is normal production of hemoglobin, along with normal maturation of red blood cells.

15. **(4)** The key in this question is "primary prevention." Iron is readily bioavailable in breast milk (this is the reason stools are yellow and pasty—most iron is absorbed and not excreted). Iron-enriched formula during the first 6 months of life helps build sufficient iron stores to deal with the "finicky" diet of the toddler.

16. **(2)** Lymphadenopathy as described, without evidence of infection, should always be referred to a surgeon for biopsy, because biopsy is the only definitive test to rule out a malignancy (a frequent cause of lymphadenopathy not caused by infectious processes). There are no signs or symptoms to suggest the need for a throat culture, monospot, or chest x-ray. Not intervening is not appropriate because the cause of lymphadenopathy needs to be determined.

17. **(3)** This constellation of symptoms (fever, night sweats, weight loss) is used in the staging of NHL; their presence is considered to be a poor prognostic indicator. The other symptoms may occur depending on the amount of disease involvement, but are not

considered "B" symptoms, also known as constitutional symptoms.

18. **(4)** Beef, spinach, and peanut butter are iron-rich foods. The remaining selection are examples of foods rich in calcium, fiber, and vitamin C, respectively.

19. **(3)** With an iron deficiency anemia, there is a reduced amount of hemoglobin, which carries oxygen. Long-term oxygen deprivation can lead to impaired cognitive and motor development. Megaloblastic anemia results from a deficiency of vitamin $B_{12}$ and/or folate intake. Crohn's disease has a familial incidence and leads to problems associated with diarrhea. The liver and spleen are both involved with red blood cell production.

20. **(4)** Sickle disease is transmitted by two parents who have the sickle cell trait; however, they do not show symptoms of the disease. Each pregnancy carries a 25% chance of sickle cell disease and 25% chance of the child carrying the trait.

21. **(3)** An iron deficiency anemia is commonly found in this age group, especially in infants who do not eat a balanced diet that includes foods rich in iron (i.e., iron-fortified cereals). This is a microcytic, hypochromic anemia with a decrease in serum iron (ferritin). The MCV would be decreased (<90).

22. **(4)** The normal full-term infant is born with sufficient iron stores to prevent iron deficiency for the first 6 months of life.

23. **(1)** The anemia of plumbism is typically microcytic, hypochromic. It is important to rule out an associated iron deficiency anemia, as it manifests as microcytic, hypochromic also. Remember, the lead affects heme synthesis by blocking the incorporation of iron into the protoporphyrin compound that makes up the heme portion of hemoglobin.

24. **(2)** Henoch-Schönlein purpura is characterized by rash, arthritis, gastrointestinal symptoms, and renal abnormalities. All of the other symptoms occur with hemophilia.

## Pharmacology

25. **(3)** Treatment of the underlying condition leads to resolution of the anemia of chronic disease. Folic acid and iron supplements are indicated for folate and iron deficiency anemias, respectively. Epoetin alfa (Epogen) injections are indicated for those conditions that affect erythropoiesis, namely chronic renal failure, chemotherapy-induced anemia, and acquired immunodeficiency syndrome.

26. **(2)** Iron medications can cause staining of the teeth, so it is a good practice to give the medication through a straw. It is best to give iron on an empty stomach (if tolerable) to increase absorption. Ascorbic acid increases absorption of iron. If a dose is missed, it is best to give the dose when it is remembered as long as it is not too close to the next dose. You would not increase the next two doses.

27. **(3)** AHF *antihemophilic factor* is stable for 24 hours at room temperature, but should be used within 1–3 hours. It should *not* be refrigerated or frozen after reconstituted and is clear and colorless or yellow. It should be gently agitated or rotated to dissolve, not vigorously shaken. It may take 5–10 minutes to completely dissolve.

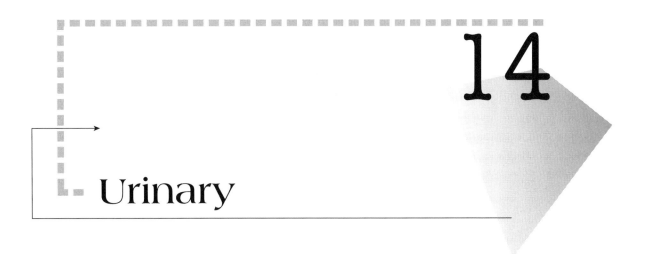

# Urinary

## Physical Examination & Diagnostic Tests

1. A urinalysis that suggests a urinary tract infection shows:

   1. Protein only.
   2. Alkaline pH and positive nitrite and leukocyte esterase.
   3. Hematuria and pyuria only.
   4. Red color without the presence of red blood cells.

2. An intravenous urography and voiding cystourethrography assists in diagnosing:

   1. Congenital anomalies, stone formation, or foreign bodies.
   2. Renal size and the presence of stone.
   3. A problem in the urethra, prostate, or bladder.
   4. Visualization of the ureter and renal pelvis.

3. Physical exam on an adolescent reveals 2+ proteinuria. The next step in differential diagnosis would involve:

↑protein excretion while in the upright position and normal protein excretion in a supine or recumbent position. common in adolescents

   1. Quantifying protein excretion.
   2. Evaluating for orthostatic proteinuria.
   3. Reassuring the patient and following up in 6 months.
   4. Evaluating for nephritis.

## Disorders

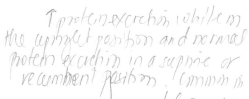

"bed wetting" urinary incontinence

4. At what age is a child considered enuretic, if he has not attained bladder control?

   1. 2 years.
   2. 3 years.
   3. 4 years.
   4. 5 years.

5. An adolescent explains to the nurse practitioner that she has been having frequent and painful urination. The nurse practitioner orders a clean-catch urine for routine urinalyis and culture and sensitivity (C&S). The laboratory C&S report is as follows: $10^5$ *Escherichia coli* and $10^4$ *Staphylococcus epidermidis* per milliliter. The nurse practitioner would: *10000·*

   1. Treat the *E. coli.*

   2. Order penicillin.

   3. Treat the *S. epidermidis.* *mostlikely contaminate*

   4. Encourage citric fruit juices.

6. A young adolescent comes to the student health clinic complaining of severe abdominal discomfort and bloody urine. Priority in the diagnostic work-up should include:

   1. Intravenous pyelogram (IVP) to rule out a kidney stone.

   2. Straining all urine.

   3. Microscopic urine exam. *for WBC*

   4. A 24-hr urine culture.

7. In children, the presence of hypertension and a history of a sore throat may be an indication of:

   1. Congestive heart failure.

   2. Glomerulonephritis.

   3. Vasculitis.

   4. Cushing's syndrome.

8. When assessing a child with glomerulonephritis, what symptoms would the nurse practitioner anticipate to be present?

   1. Fever >102°F and bilateral flank pain.

   2. Periorbital edema and increase in blood pressure.

   3. Anorexia and complaints of dysuria.

   4. Oliguria with strong, concentrated urine.

9. In considering the management of an enuretic child, the nurse practitioner understands:

   1. Imipramine (Tofranil) is the appropriate medication to prescribe.

   2. Behavior modification is the preferred method of management for enuresis.

   3. Enuresis is usually associated with some type of congenital urinary system disorder.

   4. Enuresis is characterized by repeated voiding of urine into the bed or clothes occurring at age 3 years.

10. When instructing the parents regarding the course of poststreptococcal glomerulonephritis, the nurse practitioner lets them know to expect the bloody urine for at least how many weeks after onset of diuresis?

    1. 1 week.

    2. 1–2 weeks.

    3. 2–3 weeks.

    4. 4–7 days.

11. A mother brings in her 3-year-old daughter stating she noticed a swelling in the child's abdominal area just below the rib cage on the left side. The nurse practitioner observes a bulging of the area and the child does not want to be touched due to abdominal tenderness. What is the best action for the nurse practitioner at this visit?

    1. Immediately contact a pediatrician for consultation.

    2. Schedule a referral with a pediatrician in the near future.

    3. Perform a urinalysis and draw blood for creatinine and potassium.

    4. Explain to the child it is necessary to examine the abdomen.

12. A nurse practitioner recognizes what factors as contributing to the development of pre-renal failure?

    1. History of an anaphylactic reaction that rendered the child unconscious.

    2. Extended treatment of an infection with gentamin (Garamycin).

3. Acute pyelonephritis and consequent glomerulonephritis.

4. Bilateral stricture of the ureters.

13. The nurse practitioner understands the difference between primary and secondary enuresis is:

1. Primary enuresis occurs when the child has a period of dryness and then starts bedwetting again.

2. Primary enuresis is caused by a small bladder capacity and bladder irritation.

3. Secondary enuresis involves children who have never experienced an extended period of dryness (2–3 months) without some type of treatment, such as medications.

4. Secondary enuresis primarily affects girls, usually 4 years of age, and is often associated with glomerulonephritis and other renal infections.

14. Which statement is correct regarding glomerulonephritis?

1. Hypertension and proteinuria rarely occur.

2. The client may have hematuria after exercise for up to 2 years after resolution.

3. Resolution of acute symptoms occurs in 2–3 months.

4. It affects mostly females following an acute urinary tract infection.

15. The nurse practitioner understands that burgundy red urine is a sign of which condition?

1. Congenital syphilis.

2. Congenital porphyria.

3. α-Trypsin deficiency.

4. Hepatitis.   *Tea cola*

# Pharmacology

16. A 6-year-old girl is brought to the clinic by her mother. The child is complaining of burning on urination and the urine is cloudy. A dipstick test of the urine is positive for leukocyte esterase. The mother states the child had a fever with nausea and vomiting the last time she took Gantrisin (sulfisoxazole). The medication of choice for this client is:

1. Nitrofurantoin (Macrodantin) 50 mg PO qid × 7 days.

2. Trimethoprim-sulfamethoxazole (Septra D.S.) 1 tab PO bid × 10 days.

3. Ciprofloxacin (Cipro) 200 mg PO bid × 10 days.

4. Clarithromycin (Biaxin) 250 mg PO bid × 10 days.

17. Which medication is not a drug of choice for a child experiencing acute glomerulonephritis?

1. Captopril (Capoten).

2. Furosemide (Lasix).

3. Penicillin (Pen-Vee K).

4. Tetracycline (Achromycin).

18. What is the usual PO dosage for furosemide (Lasix) in children?

1. 10–20 mg/kg.

2. 1–2 mg/kg.

3. 0.1–0.2 mg/kg.

4. 5–10 mg/kg.

# **14** Answers & Rationales

## Physical Examination & Diagnostic Tests

1. **(2)** These are results indicating the presence of a urinary tract infection. Proteinuria alone suggests glomerulonephritis. Hematuria and pyuria without bacteria may indicate chlamydia, gonorrhea, viral infection, or, less commonly, tuberculosis. If a dipstick test is negative for red blood cells but the urine color is red, a substance that can change the color of the urine is likely the cause.

2. **(1)** In an intravenous urography and voiding cystourethrography, congenital anomalies, stone formation, or foreign bodies can be identified. Renal size and the presence of stones can be seen in flat plate and upright films of the abdomen. In a cystoscopy, the urethra, prostate, and bladder can be visualized. A urethroscopy can visualize the ureter and renal pelvis.

3. **(2)** Twenty-five to 60% of proteinuria in children is orthostatic in nature and must be evaluated first.

## Disorders

4. **(4)** A child is considered enuretic if bladder control is not attained at age 5.

5. **(1)** *Escherichia coli* is the most common organism causing urinary tract infections (UTIs) in the young female. Counts of $10^5$ are diagnostic and should be treated with trimethoprim-sulfamethoxazole (Bactrim DS) or any suitable, sensitive anti-infective agent. *Staphylococcus epidermidis* is more often a contaminant due to inappropriate clean-catch specimen collection technique.

6. **(3)** The nurse practitioner suspects a urinary tract infection and needs to confirm with a microscopic urinalysis exam to identify presence of white blood cells and bacteria.

7. **(2)** Acute hypertension in children and adolescents almost always is due to an identifiable secondary cause, such as glomerulonephritis due to strep infections.

8. **(2)** The facial edema and increased blood pressure are common. Generally, the child does not have a high fever and the urine is not concentrated, but it may be decreased in amount.

9. **(2)** Pharmacologic treatment with imipramine is no longer recommended. Nonpharmacologic treatments include behavior programs such as use of a buzzer or bell system, positive reinforcement, avoiding liquids after dinner, and urinating immediately before going to bed.

10. **(2)** There can be gross hematuria for 1–2 weeks after the diuresis and microscopic hematuria for up to 2 years. If parents know what to expect, they will know what is abnormal and when to notify a health care professional.

11. **(1)** The pediatrician should be contacted immediately; this is frequently the first sign of a Wilms' tumor, which is very fragile and possibly malignant. Children should not be referred due to the chance they will not be seen immediately. A urinalysis and blood test can be done, but often these tests are negative, so the child should be seen by a pediatrician immediately regardless of the test results. The abdomen should not be examined due to the fragility of the tumor.

12. **(1)** The precipitating factor in prerenal failure is most often a hypotensive or hypoxic episode precipitated renal ischemia, most often a hypotensive situation. Nephrotoxic medications and pyelonephritis are causes of intrarenal failure. Stricture of the ureters is postrenal are all causes of intrarenal failure.

13. **(2)** Enuresis affects approximately 10% of all children (mostly boys, after age 4) and is usually caused by a small bladder capacity and irritation. Option #1 describes secondary enuresis. Option #3 describes primary enuresis. Secondary enuresis may be caused by diabetes, urinary tract and anatomic abnormalities, and psychological factors.

14. **(2)** Other outcomes include resolution of acute symptoms in 2–3 weeks, hypertension and proteinuria that may persist into adulthood, and possible development of chronic renal failure. Mostly, glomerulonephritis affects males following a group A β-hemolytic streptococcal infection (e.g., untreated impetigo, strep throat).

15. **(2)** The excretion of urine that is burgundy red is characteristic of congenital porphyria, which usually manifests shortly after birth. Tea-colored urine is characteristic of hepatitis.

# Pharmacology

16. **(1)** The clinical presentation is that of a urinary tract infection (UTI). The dipstick is positive for bacteria. Since the child may have had a reaction to a sulfa drug (Gantrisen), it would be best to avoid sulfa drugs at this time. The next best medication for a UTI in children is nitrofurantoin (Macrodantin). Ciprofloxacin is not recommended for children under 18 years old, and clarithromycin is not a first-line drug of choice for UTI.

17. **(4)** Tetracyclines are not indicated because penicillin is the drug of choice to treat β-hemolytic streptococcus. Antihypertensives (angiotensin-converting enzyme inhibitors), diuretics, and cation exchange resins (Kayexalate) are first-line therapy to deal with the symptoms.

18. **(2)** The usual PO dosage is 1–2 mg/kg q6–8h and prn.

# Male Reproductive

## Physical Examination & Diagnostic Tests

1. Which organ is **not** palpable on physical examination of an adolescent male client?

   1. Vas deferens.

   2. Testes.

   3. Epididymis.

   4. Cowper's glands. *AkA Bulbourethral gland*

2. A review of a lab report with an elevated serum gonadotropin would raise suspicion of which disorder?

   1. Seminal vesiculitis.

   2. Vas deferens disease.

   3. Testicular disease.

   4. Congenital adrenal hyperplasia.

3. Which of the following structures can be palpated during an external examination of an adolescent male client?

   1. Epididymis.

   2. Cowper's ducts.

   3. Seminal vesicles.

   4. Ejaculatory ducts.

4. What would be most helpful in diagnosing gynecomastia?

   1. History and physical examination.

   2. Liver function test.

   3. Thyroid function test.

   4. Mammogram.

5. The correct position in which to place a healthy, adolescent male client to examine the rectum and prostate is:

   1. Left lateral Sims with right knee flexed and left leg extended.

   2. Supine with hips and legs flexed and feet positioned on the examining table.

   3. Modified knee–chest with client prone and knees flexed under hips.

   4. Leaning over the examination table with chest and shoulders resting on the table.

161

6. When examining the scrotum of an adolescent Hispanic male, a normal finding is:

    1. Symmetrical scrotal sac with two movable testes.

    2. Smooth, rubbery, sac-like surface that is sensitive to gentle compression.

    3. Asymmetrical sac with the left side lower than the right side.

    4. A reddened color that is darker than body skin with sebaceous cysts.

# Disorders

7. What finding is indicative of testicular torsion?

    1. Scrotal swelling with tenderness that occurs only after age 25.

    2. Sudden onset of pain with a firm, tender mass in the scrotum.

    3. Positive Prehn's sign.

    4. Cremasteric reflex present.

8. The treatment of choice for testicular torsion by the nurse practitioner is:

    1. Massage of involved side of scrotum by the client tid with ice.

    2. Ceftriaxone (Rocephin) 500 mg bid × 4 days.

    3. Immediate surgical referral.

    4. Bed rest with elevation of the scrotum and heat alternating with ice.

9. Which statement is correct concerning circumcision?

    1. Circumcision is helpful in preventing phimosis.

    2. Circumcision is a cause of paraphimosis.

    3. Balanoposthitis is the direct result of circumcision.

    4. Circumcision increases the incidence of cancer of the penis.

10. Acute epididymitis is characterized by:

    1. Absence of dysuria.

    2. Scrotum is not enlarged.

    3. Tenderness over the epididymis.

    4. Abdominal pain is absent.

11. Which one of the following is a correct statement about hypogonadism?

    1. Usually presents with impotence.

    2. May cause an increased libido.

    3. Is not associated with gynecomastia.

    4. Does not contribute to infertility.

12. Circumcision can prevent which of the following?

    1. Paraphimosis.

    2. Epididymitis.

    3. Sexually transmitted diseases.

    4. Prostatitis.

13. Which statement is true about the prostate?

    1. Secretes fluid that is acid.

    2. Secretes fluid that is alkaline.

    3. Secretes androgens.

    4. Produces sperm.

14. A 15-year-old male presents with complaints of severe scrotal pain for the past 2 hours. The scrotum is swollen and extremely tender, so palpation of the epididymis is not possible. The nurse practitioner recognizes the immediate treatment is:

    1. Narcotic analgesics and bed rest.

    2. Warm packs and scrotal support.

    3. Antibiotics, ice packs, and analgesics.

    4. Referral to surgeon for exploration.

15. An 18-year-old male client presents with scrotal pain. A suspected diagnosis that requires immediate referral is:

    1. Testicular torsion.

    2. Hydrocele.

    3. Epididymitis.

    4. Inguinal hernia.

16. A young male client presents with a complaint of a feeling of fullness in the scrotum. Physical examination reveals a round, soft, nontender, nonadherent, bluish discolored testicular mass resembling a "bag of worms"; there is no variation in size with respiration or Valsalva maneuver. The mass transilluminates and is located anterior to the testes. The most likely diagnosis is:

    1. Varicocele.

    2. Hernia.

    3. Tumor.

    4. Spermatocele.

17. An uncircumcised adolescent presents with a complaint of not being able to retract the foreskin over the glans penis. The most likely diagnosis is:

    1. Lateral phimosis.

    2. Phimosis.

    3. Peyronie's disease.

    4. Paraphimosis.

18. An adolescent is diagnosed with balanitis; the most likely cause is:

    1. Candidiasis.

    2. Herpes genitalis.

    3. Lichen planus.

    4. Psoriasis.

19. An adolescent presents with a complaint of dysuria, enlarged scrotal tenderness over the epididymis, and abdominal pain. The most likely diagnosis is:

    1. Testicular torsion.

    2. Vas deferens inflammation.

    3. Epididymitis.

    4. Balanitis.

20. On a routine physical examination an adolescent expresses concern over the observation that one side of his scrotum is larger than the other. He states it has been getting larger for the past few months; the scrotum is smaller in the morning and gets larger through the day. He has felt a heaviness in the scrotum, denies any acute pain but does confirm some discomfort in his lower back. He denies any history of trauma to the scrotal area. On examination the nurse practitioner confirms the enlargement, and on further examination determines the scrotum will transilluminate and manual manipulation of the scrotum does not cause pain. The initial diagnosis for this adolescent is:

    1. Hydrocele.

    2. Orchitis.

    3. Epididymitis.

    4. Traumatic injury.

21. The nurse practitioner understands that idiopathic scrotal edema:

    1. Is a self-limiting process characterized by erythema, edema, and mild tenderness of the scrotal wall.

    2. Occurs in older adolescents, often precipitated by a sports injury.

    3. Is a chronic process characterized by scrotal edema, testicular atrophy, and moderate pain and tenderness.

    4. Occurs in conjunction with a varicocele.

22. Concerning the male breast, which is a correct statement?

    1. Gynecomastia is the result of low estrogen and normal levels of testosterone.

    2. Most breast cancers in men are estrogen-receptor positive.

    3. Breast cancer is males is very common.

    4. Gynecomastia is a nonhormonal or tissue alteration.

23. Which statement is correct concerning testicular cancer?

    1. Rarely occurs in boys with a history of undescended testes.

    2. This problem is directly related to testicular trauma.

    3. Testicular cancer presents suddenly with pain.

    4. Testicular cancer is primarily found in young males.

24. Which finding is indicative of orchitis?

    1. Extremely painful scrotum.

    2. No history of parotitis.

    3. No evidence of systemic viral infection.

    4. Decreased serum amylase.

25. An adolescent has nongonococcal urethritis (NGU). The nurse practitioner understands that:

    1. No related problems occur if untreated.

    2. It is often asymptomatic.

    3. It is easily differentiated from gonococcal urethritis on physical examination.

    4. There is a very purulent discharge with a foul odor.

26. What organism is the most common cause of NGU in males?

    1. *Chlamydia trachomatis*.

    2. *Neisseria gonorrhoeae*.

    3. *Escherichia coli*.

    4. *Streptococcus faecalis*.

27. Cryptorchidism is defined as:

    1. Testicular underdevelopment.

    2. Imbalance of estrogen–androgen ratio.

    3. Undescended testicles.

    4. Absence of spermatogenesis.

28. The causative agent of orchitis is:

    1. Arbovirus.

    2. Echovirus.

    3. Mumps.

    4. Rubeola.

29. A 14-year-old boy comes into the clinic from school with complaints of severe scrotal pain radiating inguinally that began suddenly. He is experiencing no difficulty voiding and has some nausea but no vomiting. Examination reveals scrotal edema and erythema; the scrotum on the affected side is slightly higher than the unaffected side, and the cremasteric reflex is negative. The nurse practitioner determines the best treatment for this client is:

    1. Bed rest with ice pack and scrotal elevation.

    2. Warm scrotal pack and return to clinic the next day.

    3. Immediate referral to a urologist.

    4. Schedule for an ultrasound in the morning.

30. A 18-year-old client with a history of sickle cell disease complains of a sudden problem with erections that are not sexually oriented. He is currently experiencing a painful erection and he is unable to void. The nurse practitioner determines the treatment of choice is:

    1. Meperidine (Demerol) and bed rest.

    2. Immediate referral to a urologist.

    3. Increase hydration for sickle cell crisis.

    4. Determine level of testosterone.

31. The nurse practitioner is speaking with a group of male teenagers. They are most concerned about symptoms associated with gonorrhea. The nurse practitioner discusses with them:

    1. There may be reddish lesions on the palms of the hands and soles of the feet.

    2. Men may observe a rash over the body of the penis.

    3. Urinary dribbling may occur due to the irritation of the urinary tract.

    4. Painful urination occurs due to the inflammation of the urethra.

# Pharmacology

32. In planning the treatment for a client with balanitis, the nurse practitioner orders:

    1. Rest, ice, and elevation.

    2. Massage.

    3. Antifungals.

    4. Emergency circumcision.

33. A young adolescent complains of scrotal pain with dysuria and frequency that has been increasing over the past two weeks. Physical examination reveals extreme tenderness and swelling of the scrotum, there is a urethral discharge, the testes are normal in size and position. A urinalysis reveals pyuria; culture positive for chlamydia. What is an appropriate prescription to write?

   1. Nitrofurantoin (Macrodantin) 100 mg PO qid × 14 days.

   2. Doxycycline (Vibramycin) 100 mg PO bid × 10 days.

   3. Metrondiazole (Flagyl) 250 mg PO tid × 7 days.

   4. Oxbutynin (Ditropan) 5 mg PO tid × 10 days.

34. A sexually active adolescent complains of purulent urethral discharge and dysuria for the past 2 days. Urethral culture is positive for gonococcus, negative chlamydia. The medication of choice is:

   1. Ceftrixone (Rocephin) 500 mg IM followed by 7 days of doxycycline 100 mg PO bid.

   2. Penicillin G (Bicillin) 2.4 million units IM followed by 7 days of penicillin V (Pen-Vee K) 500 mg tid.

   3. Metrondiazole (Flagyl) 250 mg PO tid × 7 days.

   4. TMP-SMZ (Septra D.S.) 1 tab PO bid × 10 days.

# 15 Answers & Rationales

## Physical Examination & Diagnostic Tests

1. **(4)** Cowper's glands (bulbourethral glands) are located near the prostate and beside the urethra near the base of the penis. These glands are part of the internal and nonpalpable genitalia that consist of glands and ducts. The testes, vas deferens, and epididymis are part of the external genitalia.

2. **(3)** Gonadotropin is elevated in testicular disease. Congenital adrenal hyperplasia results in inadequate serum cortisol and an oversecretion of sex steroids.

3. **(1)** The epididymis is part of the external genitalia, while the ducts and glands are part of the internal genitalia. The epididymis is palpated on the posterolateral surface of each testis and is a comma-shaped structure. The seminal vesicles (pair of glands) lie behind the urinary bladder in front of the rectum. These vesicles join the ampulla of the vas deferens to form the ejaculatory duct.

4. **(1)** A complete history and physical will usually provide the cause of gynecomastia without further testing, since it can be caused by medication, starving and refeeding, or lack of androgen production (atrophying testes), which changes the estrogen–androgen ratio.

5. **(4)** For client comfort and ease of examination, the healthy, ambulatory adolescent client is asked to lean over the examination table with his chest and upper body resting on the table. Although Option #1 is correct, it is the position used for examining a client who is confined to the bed.

6. **(3)** The scrotal sac is asymmetrical with the left side lower than right side. It is darker than body skin, and often appears reddened in red-haired men (abnormal finding if found in clients without red hair, i.e., Hispanic male). It has a surface that may be coarse with small lumps on the skin, which are sebaceous or epidermoid cysts that may have an oily discharge.

## Disorders

7. **(2)** Sudden onset of pain with a firm, tender mass in the scrotum is indicative of testicular torsion; the pain is not relieved when the involved testicle is elevated to relieve pressure. Prehn's sign (passive elevation of the testis may relieve pain) is associated with epididymitis. The cremasteric reflex is absent. Testicular torsion is most common among neonates and adolescents, with highest incidence at time of puberty.

8. **(3)** Immediate surgical referral is necessary and should be done within 6 hours postsymptoms to preserve normal testicular function. The other treatments listed are indicated in epididymitis.

9. **(1)** Circumcision is helpful in preventing phimosis and paraphimosis as both are retraction dysfunctions of the prepuce. In phimosis, the foreskin is too tight to be retracted backward over the glans penis. In paraphimosis, once the foreskin has been retracted behind the glans penis, it is too constricted to return to a position of covering the glans penis. Balanoposthitis is an inflammation of the glans penis and prepuce.

10. **(3)** Acute epididymitis is characterized by an acute scrotal pain, dysuria, and enlarged unilateral scrotum with abdominal pain. Scrotal pain is relieved when the involved testicle is elevated.

11. **(1)** A male will present with impotence and decreased libido. These same clients will often have gynecomastia due to the low or absent production of gonadotropin. Klinefelter's syndrome (a chromosomal abnormality with a karyotype of 47,XXY–47,XXXXY) is the most common cause of male hypogonadism, with failure of both spermatic function and virilization.

12. **(1)** Paraphimosis is a retraction disorder related to a constricted prepuce that can be relieved through circumcision.

13. **(2)** The prostate secretes fluid that is alkaline and helps sperm survive in the acid environment of the female reproductive tract. Androgens are produced by the Leydig cells of the testes. Sperm are produced in the seminiferous tubules of the testes.

14. **(4)** This involves the differential diagnosis between epididymitis and testicular torsion. Irreversible damage will be done to the testicles if torsion is not released within 3–4 hours. Time should not be wasted with other treatments if torsion is strongly suspected.

15. **(1)** Testicular torsion and testicular cancer are considerations that are potentially curable but must be treated early. Hydrocele, epididymitis, and inguinal hernias also require referrals but do not require immediate attention.

16. **(1)** Varicocele presents as described, whereas a hernia may transilluminate and sometimes bowel sounds can be auscultated in the scrotum. Hernias vary in size with Valsalva maneuvers. Tumors do not transilluminate.

17. **(2)** Phimosis is a retraction disorder of the penile foreskin or prepuce and can occur at any age; it is usually the result of poor hygiene and chronic infection (the foreskin cannot be retracted back over the glans penis). Peyronie's disease is a fibrotic condition that causes lateral curvature of the penis during erection. Paraphimosis is the inability to retract the foreskin from behind the glans penis.

18. **(1)** Candidiasis is the usual cause for balanitis, which is inflammation of the glans penis and prepuce usually associated with poor hygiene. Balanitis is usually found in an adolescent male with poorly controlled diabetes and candidiasis.

19. **(3)** Epididymitis presents as described, and on palpation the epididymis will often feel like a bag of worms in the scrotal sac rather than a fairly smooth cord.

20. **(1)** The lack of pain, increase in size of scrotal contents, and transillumination are characteristic of hydrocele. Orchitis and epididymitis are usually characterized by pain; orchitis most often is associated with parotitis or mumps. There is no history of injury and the scrotum would be tender to palpation.

21. **(1)** Idiopathic (etiology unknown) scrotal edema is a self-limiting process characterized by erythema, edema, and mild tenderness of the scrotal wall. It may occur at any age from 18 months to 14 years. It resolves spontaneously and is not associated with a varicocele (dilated veins of the pampiniform plexus).

22. **(2)** Gynecomastia is the result of an increased estrogen-to-androgen ratio in males; as a result their breast cancers are receptor positive.

23. **(4)** Testicular cancer is primarily found in young men and presents as nonpainful nodules of the involved testicle. Trauma is not a causal factor. It is 20–40 times more common in boys with undescended testes.

24. **(1)** Usually orchitis presents with a tender, unilaterally swollen testicle within 7–10 days of mumps (parotitis). An elevated serum amylase is associated with inflammation of the salivary glands (i.e., mumps).

25. **(2)** NGU is often asymptomatic and as such is difficult to diagnose. NGU commonly has a clear discharge and is usually caused by chlamydia. Gonococcal urethritis usually produces a yellow, purulent discharge. If there is a discharge with NGU, it is hard to differentiate from gonorrhea without a culture. Reiter's syndrome is also associated with untreated chlamydia infections of the urogenital tract.

26. **(1)** *Chlamydia trachomatis* is the most common organism in males with NGU.

27. **(3)** Cryptorchidism is the result of undescended testes, either bilateral or, more often, affecting the right testis. Normally, descent occurs in the seventh to eighth month of gestation.

28. **(3)** The mumps virus is responsible for causing orchitis. Arbovirus and echovirus are implicated in meningitis/encephalitis. Rubeola is associated with complications of otitis media, pneumonia, croup, and encephalitis.

29. **(3)** The symptoms described are consistent with testicular torsion. This is an emergent surgical problem, and the client should be referred immediately.

30. **(2)** This is considered a urologic emergency because the circulation to the penis may be compromised, as well as because of the inability to void. The client should be referred immediately to a physician.

31. **(4)** Dysuria is one of the most common complaints of young men with gonorrhea. There are no lesions, rash, or urinary dribbling along with the yellow discharge.

# Pharmacology

32. **(3)** Antifungals (e.g., topical nystatin [Mycostatin] or Ciclopirox [Loprox]) are the treatment of choice. If the infection is recalcitrant, give oral fluconazole (Diflucan) 150 mg/day or itraconazole (Sporanox) 100 mg/day. All the other treatments are inappropriate.

33. **(2)** The adolescent is presenting with classic symptoms of epididymitis due to chlamydia. The treatment of choice is doxycycline (Vibramycin) 100 mg PO bid × 10 days. Nitrofurantoin is a urinary antiseptic and oxbutynin is indicated for incontinence or enuresis. On differential diagnosis the gradual onset of pain, voiding problems, urethral discharge, and swelling are more indicative of epididymitis then testicular torsion.

34. **(1)** This is the recommended treatment for uncomplicated gonorrhea infection in an adolescent. Ceftrixone (Rocephin) 500 mg IM followed by 7 days of doxycycline (Vibramycin) 100 mg PO bid or tetracycline (Achromycin) 500 mg PO qid × 7 days.

# 16

## Female Reproductive

## Physical Examination & Diagnostic Tests

1. When obtaining a cervical specimen for a Pap smear, the nurse practitioner:

    1. Lubricates the speculum with a water-soluble lubricant to assist in the insertion of the instrument.

    2. Utilizes the cervical brush when obtaining the cervical cells on a prenatal client due to the presence of the cervical mucous plug.

    3. Uses warm water to lubricate the speculum to assist in the insertion of the instrument.

    4. Completes the bimanual portion of the exam first in order to determine the relative position of the cervix to assist in a comfortable insertion of the speculum.

2. To promote client comfort prior to performing a pelvic exam, the nurse practitioner:

    1. Asks the client to bear down slightly as the speculum is inserted.

    2. Has the client empty her bladder.

    3. Explains each step of the procedure in a calm manner.

    4. Carefully reassures the client that the exam will only take a few minutes.

3. What finding is considered a normal surface characteristic of the cervix?

    1. Small, yellow, raised round area on cervix.

    2. Red patchy areas with occasional white spots.

    3. Friable, bleeding tissue at opening of cervical os.

    4. Irregular, granular surface with red patches.

4. The primary role of a breast ultrasound is:

    1. Screening test for breast cancer.

    2. Used for definitive diagnosis of breast cancer.

    3. Used to determine if a breast lesion is cystic or solid.

    4. Used to locate small lesions prior to surgery.

5. Potassium hydroxide (KOH) use when doing a wet mount assists in the diagnosis of:

   1. Bacterial vaginosis and *Candida* vaginitis.

   2. *Trichomonas* and chlamydia.

   3. Syphilis and gonorrhea.

   4. Herpes and condyloma.

6. The nurse practitioner is reviewing the lab results of an 18-year-old client seen recently for a Pap smear. The results are as follows: Classification—high-grade squamous intraepithelial lesion; endocervical cells seen; adequate smear. The nurse practitioner phones the client and tells her which of the following?

   1. "Your Pap smear was normal. Follow up in 1 year, sooner if problems arise."

   2. "Your Pap smear shows invasive cancer. I would like you to see a gynecologic oncologist for treatment."

   3. "Your Pap smear shows abnormal tissue that needs to be evaluated. Please schedule an appointment for a colposcopy."

   4. "Your Pap smear shows a minor abnormality. Sometimes this can signify a disease process just beginning. Please schedule another Pap smear in 4 months for follow-up."

7. When describing the findings from a normal breast examination in an 18-year-old female, the nurse practitioner documents on the client record:

   1. Left nipple everted, several coarse black hairs arising from the areola, enlarged axillary lymph nodes palpated bilaterally, and tender nodes in supraclavicular area.

   2. No dimpling or retraction; 1-cm hard, fixed, stellate mass noted next to nipple with scant nipple discharge; no pain or tenderness on palpation.

   3. Right breast slightly larger and denser than left with no nipple discharge, right areola dark pink in color and inverted, left areola dark brown in color and everted, breasts tender to palpation with no axillary nodes noted.

   4. Pendulous breasts with no dimpling, retraction, nipple discharge, or areas of discoloration; numerous small nevi near areola with Montgomery tubercles noted; no supraclavicular or axillary lymph nodes palpated.

8. Which test is the "gold standard" for the diagnosis of chlamydia?

   1. Use of KOH wet mount "whiff" test.

   2. Presence of inflammatory cells in Pap smear.

   3. Direct fluorescent antibody (DFA).

   4. Culture with special media and collection technique.

9. Which is the most accurate statement regarding a reactive serologic test for syphilis?

   1. All reactive serologic tests require confirmation with a treponemal test.

   2. Reactive serologic tests are highly suspicious for active syphilis.

   3. A false-positive serologic test, though rare, can be unnecessarily traumatizing to a client.

   4. A reactive serologic test most likely implies the need for retreatment.

10. While working up an older adolescent with secondary amenorrhea, the prolactin serum assay results show a level of 24 ng/ml. Appropriate management includes:

   1. Administering medroxyprogesterone acetate 10 mg bid × 5 days.

   2. Referring to an endocrinologist.

   3. Recording the results as within normal limits.

   4. Assessing for nipple discharge.

11. When evaluating a young adult with amenorrhea and normal secondary sex characteristics, the purpose of the progesterone challenge is to determine the presence of:

   1. Endogenous estrogen.

2. Thyroxine.

3. Prolactin.

4. Adequate body fat.

12. What is the most important information in the history that will assist the nurse practitioner who is trying to establish a diagnosis of premenstrual syndrome (PMS) in an adolescent with complaints for the past four menstrual cycles of fatigue, breast tenderness, abdominal bloating, fluid retention, irritability, and difficulty sleeping the week before the onset of menses?

1. Occurrence of symptoms in the menstrual cycle.

2. Severity of the symptoms.

3. Number and frequency over past 4 months.

4. Presence or absence of anxiety or depression.

# Normal Gynecology

13. The nurse practitioner understands that PMS occurs with greatest frequency and severity in the:

1. Late luteal phase.

2. Follicular phase.

3. Proliferative phase.

4. Ovulatory phase.

14. The primary function of follicle-stimulating hormone (FSH) is:

1. Stimulate maturation of ovarian follicles.

2. Promote milk secretion.

3. Trigger ovulation.

4. Inhibit release of luteinizing hormone (LH) from the pituitary gland.

15. A young woman complains to the nurse practitioner that she is experiencing headaches, irritability, decreased appetite, and fatigue for about 1 week prior to her menses. Appropriate management includes:

1. Treating the PMS with increased protein and salt in the diet.

2. Incorporating daily regular aerobic exercise into her lifestyle.

3. Ordering a complete blood count (CBC), SMAC 12, and urinalysis.

4. Supplementing the diet with an additional 1–2 gm of vitamin C.

16. While assessing a 16-year-old girl, the nurse practitioner was asked about douching. What information would be used in the nurse practitioner's teaching plan?

1. Douching during menstruation is safe.

2. Due to vaginal discharge, daily douching is important.

3. Hypoallergenic douches include flavored or perfumed types.

4. Douching removes natural mucus and upsets normal vaginal flora.

# Gynecologic Disorders

17. The nurse practitioner is talking with a young adolescent who has been diagnosed with herpes simplex type 2 (genital). In discussing her care, it would be important for the nurse practitioner to include what information?

1. The initial lesions are usually worse than lesions that occur with outbreaks at a later time.

2. Her sexual partner will not contract it if she does not have sex when the lesions are present.

3. This condition can be treated and cured if she takes all of the antibiotics for 2 weeks.

4. If in the future she becomes pregnant, she will have to have a cesarean delivery.

18. The definition of bacterial vaginosis is:

    1. A syndrome resulting from homeostatic disruption in the vagina.

    2. Vaginitis caused by a flagellated protozoan.

    3. A bacterial sexually transmitted disease (STD) that can be symptomatic or asymptomatic.

    4. A virus characterized by recurrent outbreaks and remissions.

19. A 16-year-old sexually active client complains of severe dysmenorrhea. Her gynecologic exam is normal. Which management protocol is preferred?

    1. Assess for contraceptive interest and, if interested, suggest use of oral contraceptives (OCs).

    2. Suggest use of prostaglandin synthetase inhibitor (PGSI).

    3. Suggest over-the-counter use of ibuprofen.

    4. Assess exercise patterns and use of relaxation techniques.

20. Which is **not** a criterion for the diagnosis of bacterial vaginosis?

    1. Positive amine test (whiff test).

    2. Presence of clue cells.

    3. Vaginal ph > 4.5.

    4. The presence of pseudohyphae.

21. The most common cause of dysfunctional uterine bleeding is:

    1. Thyroid disorder.

    2. Blood dyscrasia.

    3. Anovulation.

    4. Uterine tumor.

22. A 19-year-old female presents with scant pubic hair, minimal breast development, absent cervix, and uterus with a history of 46,XY karyotype. Your diagnosis is:

    1. Turner's syndrome.

    2. Müllerian agenesis.

    3. Testicular feminization.

    4. Gonadal dysgenesis.

23. The most common cause of a breast mass in clients ages 15–25 is:

    1. Fibroadenoma.

    2. Intraductal papilloma.

    3. Infiltrating lobular carcinoma.

    4. Fibrocystic breast syndrome.

24. An effective treatment for primary dysmenorrhea is:

    1. Nonsteroidal anti-inflammatory analgesics.

    2. Tranquilizers.

    3. Progestins.

    4. Steroids.

25. What is a cause of secondary amenorrhea?

    1. Testicular feminization.

    2. Hypogonadotropic hypogonadism.

    3. Congenital absence of uterus.

    4. Extreme exercise.

26. An older sexually active adolescent comes to the clinic. She states that about 3 weeks ago she had a sore on her labia that went away. It was not particularly painful and did not itch, and there did not seem to be any residual problems from it. The nurse practitioner treats this client by:

    1. Ordering the treponemal-specific test (FTA-ABS).

    2. Swabbing the area of the lesion for a viral culture.

    3. Advising her to notify her sexual contacts to determine if they have had any symptoms.

    4. Ordering nystatin (Mycostatin) cream to be applied to the area three to four times a day.

27. A high-school athlete presents to the clinic with concerns regarding her menstrual periods. She states she has not had a period in the past 2 months. She has been in

training and running about 3 miles a day for the past 3 months. She has lost approximately 15 lb. Her height is about 5 feet 3 inches and she currently weighs 100 lb. The best response by the nurse practitioner is to:

1. Determine the client's percentage of body fat and body mass.

2. Obtain serum FSH levels.

3. Determine serum levels of human chorionic gonadotropin (hCG).

4. Order thyroid function tests.

28. Which is **not** a risk factor for the development of cervical cancer?

    1. Human papillomavirus (HPV).

    2. Virginal status.

    3. Multiple sexual partners.

    4. Previous high-grade squamous intraepithelial lesion (HSIL).

29. An adolescent is complaining of tenderness and burning of her vulva. On examination, the vulva is edematous and excoriated. The nurse practitioner performs a wet mount prep of the vaginal secretions. It reveals pseudohyphae and spores. The diagnosis for this client is:

    1. Vulvovaginal candidiasis.

    2. *Chlamydia trachomatis*.

    3. Bacterial vaginosis.

    4. Gonorrhea.

30. The nurse practitioner understands that vaginal bleeding in prepubertal girls:

    1. Affects the hypothalmic-pituitary-ovarian axis.

    2. Reflects a localized problem in the vagina or uterus.

    3. Is associated with pregnancy complications.

    4. Is associated with endometrial polyps.

31. An 18-year-old presents to urgent care with new onset of painful sores in the vulva. These erupted yesterday and are associated with exquisite pain, fever, and flu-like symptoms of headache, general body aches, and mild dysuria. The examination reveals vesicular lesions covering the labium; extreme tenderness to palpation of the external genitalia; normal Bartholin's, Skene's, and urethral glands; normal vaginal inspection with a mild leukorrhea; normal cervical mucosa; and slightly tender, minimally enlarged inguinal lymph nodes bilaterally. What is the likely diagnosis?

    1. Gonorrhea.

    2. Chlamydia.

    3. Herpes simplex virus.

    4. Lymphogranuloma venereum.

32. A 17-year-old female client is seen for her annual exam. She is sexually active, rarely uses condoms for STD prevention, and has multiple sexual partners. She smokes one pack per day, admits to a sedentary lifestyle, and eats two meals per day, most often at fast food restaurants. Her exam is negative for any abnormality. Her family history and personal medical history are negative for major disease. There are no menstrual abnormalities; her last menstrual period (LMP) was 1 week ago. The nurse practitioner has done her Pap smear. Which would **not** be appropriate for this client?

    1. Cultures for gonorrhea and chlamydia.

    2. Lab testing: glucose, CBC with differential, and TSH.

    3. Human immunodeficiency virus (HIV) titer and rapid plasma reagin (RPR).

    4. Counseling on safe sex practice and contraceptive information.

33. A 19-year-old female client presents for her first well-woman exam; she is not sexually active and never has been. Her family history and past medical history are negative for any gynecologic diseases. Her menses occur every 28 days, lasting 5 days with a relatively moderate flow and no significant abdominal cramps. Her physical exam/visit today should include which tests?

    1. Pap smear.

    2. Cultures for gonorrhea and chlamydia.

    3. Stool hemoccult.

    4. Baseline mammogram.

34. During a gynecologic exam at the family planning clinic, an underweight 17-year-old presents with bruising around her upper torso and genitalia. She is minimally interactive and avoids eye contact as much as possible. Priority intervention should focus on:

    1. Lab work to rule out bleeding disorder.

    2. Nutritional assessment to determine possible anemia.

    3. Determination of possible physical abuse.

    4. Finding out if she has a support system.

35. Reactive cellular changes noted on a Pap smear are most often associated with:

    1. Inflammation.

    2. Use of estrogen vaginal cream.

    3. Drying artifact.

    4. Use of oral contraceptives.

36. Risk factors for cervical disease include:

    1. Delayed puberty.

    2. Viral exposure.

    3. Sexual activity after age 18 years.

    4. Contraceptive use.

37. During a breast exam on a young adolescent female, a 2-cm painless, lobular mass in the right breast that is firm and freely mobile is noted on palpation. Appropriate management includes:

    1. Continued observation and re-checking in 3 months.

    2. Referral for a mammogram.

    3. Referral for probable surgical excision.

    4. Detailed family history to determine breast cancer risk.

38. A 15-year-old female client comes to the nurse practitioner's office with a complaint of 1 day of fever of 102°F, a diffuse macular rash, vomiting, headache, and decreased urinary output. The history obtained by the nurse practitioner must include:

    1. Whether the client's immunizations are up to date.

    2. If the client is currently menstruating.

    3. If the client has a history of tuberculosis.

    4. What type of contraception the client uses.

39. A young adolescent female client presents with a history of vaginal itching and heavy white discharge. The client gives a history of no sexual activity. On exam, the nurse practitioner finds a red, edematous vulva and white patches on the vaginal walls. There is no odor to the discharge. The nurse practitioner expects what factors in the client's history?

    1. A vegetarian diet.

    2. Recent diarrhea.

    3. Poor hygiene.

    4. Recent antibiotic use.

40. A 16-year-old client comes to the office complaining of vaginal bleeding. The client states that she has used five tampons in the past 3 hours. She admits to sexual activity and takes oral contraceptives. On further questioning, the client states that she started her last pack of contraceptives "about 2 weeks late." The nurse practitioner should:

    1. Perform a STAT urine pregnancy test.

    2. Perform a STAT CBC.

    3. Discuss proper use of oral contraceptives.

    4. Send the client for a pelvic sonogram.

# Pharmacology

41. A 15-year-old female client presents to the office with complaints of dysuria, urinary frequency, and urgency. These symptoms began early this morning. She leaves a clean-catch midstream urine specimen that shows too-numerous-to-count (TNTC) white blood cells (WBC)/high-power field (HPF), four to five red blood cells/HPF, and positive nitrites. A urine culture is set up and will be ready in 3 days. Which is **not** a correct treatment for an uncomplicated lower urinary tract infection?

1. Phenazopyridine (Pyridium) 200 mg, 1 tab PO tid × 2 days.

2. Trimethoprim-sulfamethoxazole (Bactrim) DS, 1 tab PO bid × 5 days.

3. Ceftriaxone (Rocephin) 1 gm IM.

4. Nitrofurantoin (Macrobid) 1 tab PO bid × 5 days.

42. A 19-year-old female client is being seen in the clinic by the nurse practitioner. She was last seen 2 weeks ago for an upper respiratory tract infection and was treated with amoxicillin (Amoxil) 250 mg PO tid × 10 days. She completed her medication last week but now is aware of vaginal itching and a cottage cheese–like vaginal discharge. She states that she has never experienced such intense itching before. She is not on any medications and has no known drug allergies. Your treatment for this problem is:

1. Metronidazole (Flagyl) 500 mg PO bid × 7 days.

2. Clindamycin (Cleocin) vaginal cream, 1 applicator-full vaginally qHS × 7 days.

3. Fluconazole (Diflucan) 150 mg, 1 tab PO one time.

4. Hydrocortisone (Cortaid) 1% cream apply sparingly bid × 7 days.

43. A 17-year-old female client presents with complaints of a malodorous vaginal discharge described as white and watery. She and her boyfriend have been sexually active for 2 years, using condoms for STD prevention with every act of coitus. Her LMP was 1 week ago, and there are no noted changes in her normal menstrual pattern. Her wet mount with KOH results show a positive whiff test, TNTC clue cells/HPF, no lactobacilli, no hyphae or spores, no trichamonads, and few WBCs. Treatment for this client is:

1. Doxycycline (Vibratabs) 100 mg PO bid × 10 days.

2. Terconazole (Terazol 7 cream) 1 applicator-full per vagina qHS × 7 days.

3. Acyclovir (Zovirax) 200 mg, 1 PO q4h × 5 days.

4. Metronidazole (Metrogel) vaginal cream, 1 applicator-full per vagina qHS × 5 days.

44. An adolescent female is seen in the STD clinic. She noticed some itchy bumps in the vulvar area and is concerned that they could be cancer. On careful inspection the nurse practitioner notes the following: five cauliflower-like warty, pinkish colored lesions in the lower introitus; two smaller lesions nestled anteriorly to the hymenal ring of the vagina and cervix fail to reveal any abnormalities. A wet mount with KOH is negative. A culture for gonorrhea and chlamydia was obtained, a Pap smear done, and HIV titer and RPR drawn. Which is **not** an appropriate treatment for this client?

1. Podophyllin (Podoben) application; wash off in 6 hours with soap and water.

2. Trichloroacetic acid application; do not wash off.

3. Cyrotherapy with liquid nitrogen to lesions.

4. Benzathine penicillin 2.4 million units IM weekly × 3 weeks.

45. The treatment of choice for trichomoniasis is:

1. Azithromycin (Zithromax) 1 gm PO, single dose.

2. Ofloxacin (Floxin) 500 mg PO, single dose.

3. Metronidazole (Flagyl) 2 gm PO, single dose.

4. Clindamycin (Cleocin) 300 mg PO, single dose.

46. A 15-year-old adolescent comes into the office with complaints of profuse malodorous discharge. The nurse practitioner's diagnosis is bacterial vaginosis. The nurse practitioner would:

1. Advise the client to notify her sexual contacts regarding the diagnosis.

2. Treat the problem with metronidazole (Flagyl) 2 gm as one dose.

3. Initiate treatment with doxycycline (Vibramycin) 100 mg PO bid × 7 days.

4. Determine the presence of pregnancy prior to initiating a course of treatment.

47. An adolescent who is taking a low-dose OC calls the clinic in a panic stating that she forgot her pill 2 days ago. She is taking phenytoin (Dilantin) for seizure activity and has been seizure-free for over a year. "What should I do about my pills?" The most appropriate response should be:

1. Advise her to take the forgotten dose today along with the regular dose.

2. Refer her to her physician for advice about the Dilantin.

3. Advise her to continue pills, but to use another contraceptive through the rest of this cycle.

4. Advise her to come to the clinic for a "morning-after" pill.

48. A young adult female presents to the office for evaluation of abdominal pain. The client admits to recent sexual activity and states that she does not have her partner use condoms. On exam, the nurse practitioner finds vaginal discharge and cervical motion tenderness. Other than sending cultures to the lab, the nurse practitioner would treat this client with:

1. Penicillin G 2.4 million units IM.

2. Metronidazole (Flagyl) 500 mg PO bid × 7 days.

3. Ceftriaxone (Rocephin) 125 mg IM and azithromycin (Zithromax) 1 gm PO.

4. Acyclovir (Zovirax) 400 mg PO bid × 7 days.

# 16   Answers & Rationales

## Physical Examination & Diagnostic Tests

1. **(3)** Lubricants, such as Vaseline or K-Y gel, should not be used if a cervical specimen is being obtained for analysis. The cervical brush should not be used on pregnant clients. The bimanual exam is performed after the internal vaginal exam.

2. **(2)** To aid in the examination, an empty bladder will provide for client comfort and will assist the nurse practitioner in making a more accurate assessment during the bimanual portion of the exam. Options #1 and #3 help reduce the client's anxiety, which ultimately may assist in the achievement of comfort.

3. **(1)** A nabothian cyst is a small, white or yellow, raised round area on the cervix. The surface of the cervix should be smooth and may have a symmetrical, reddened circle around the os (squamocolumnar epithelium). The other options are all unexpected, abnormal findings.

4. **(3)** A breast ultrasound is used to determine if a lesion is solid or cystic. Ultrasound misses 50% of lesions less than 2 cm. The test is not sensitive enough to be used for routine screening and cannot replace mammography. The definitive diagnosis of breast cancer is the breast biopsy.

5. **(1)** KOH lyses epithelial and white blood cells, making it easier to visualize *Candida* (yeast). *Candida* cells are resistant and remain intact. KOH also assists with diagnosing bacterial vaginosis by alkalinizing vaginal discharge, causing a distinct fishy odor. This is a positive amine or whiff test.

6. **(3)** The Pap smear is a screening test for cervical cancer and precancerous states. The results of this test are clearly abnormal and must be acted upon. Waiting a year could be deleterious to the client's health. This is not the Pap smear report that one would choose to redo in 4 months; the client needs a diagnostic test, not another screening test. The diagnostic test needed to confirm the diagnosis of a high-grade lesion is the colposcopy with guided biopsies. This is not a diagnosis of cervical cancer on this Pap smear; therefore, a referral to a gynecologic oncologist is premature at this juncture.

7. **(4)** In Option #1, the abnormal finding is the enlarged lymph nodes. In Option #2, the abnormal finding is the fixed, stellate mass with nipple discharge. In Option #3, the asymmetrical size is normal but not the different colors of the areola and unilateral nipple inversion. The long-standing nevi and Montgomery tubercles in Option #4 are normal.

8. **(4)** Culture and DFA are both used. Culture is the only certain or definitive method of diagnosis. It is performed on a collected cervical specimen, it takes about 2–6 days to obtain the results. The DFA is fast and has good sensitivity and specificity.

9. **(1)** Serologic tests are good screening tests, but positive results require following up with a treponemal test to detect specific antibodies.

10. **(2)** Serum prolactin assay levels above 20 ng/ml indicate need for medical referral, usually to an endocrinologist. The most common cause of hyperprolactinemia and galactorrhea (milky breast discharge) is a pituitary tumor or lesion of the hypothalamus. Other causes may be hypothyroidism, medications (narcotics, tranquilizers, antihypertensives), and OCs.

11. **(1)** The initial work-up for this client includes determining the prolactin level by evaluating serum concentrations and determining the presence of endogenous estrogen. If the woman experiences withdrawal bleeding after the administration of oral or IM progesterone and the prolactin level is normal, this woman is producing estrogen and can be considered anovulatory. Absence of withdrawal bleeding with normal prolactin level requires further work-up.

12. **(1)** The occurrence of the symptoms during the menstrual cycle will assist the nurse practitioner to make a diagnosis of PMS. The adolescent should keep track on a calendar as to when each symptom occurs and disappears, and the onset and completion of menstrual flow.

## Normal Gynecology

13. **(1)** PMS occurs approximately 5–11 days prior to the onset of menses (late luteal phase) and is gone within 1–2 days of the onset of menses. This phase is progesterone dominant. The follicular phase is estrogen dominant.

14. **(1)** FSH stimulates the maturation of ovarian follicles, resulting in a dominant follicle. Milk secretion is dependent on prolactin. The production and release of LH is regulated by estrogen. LH is responsible for ovulation.

15. **(2)** Conservative management for PMS includes daily exercise, support and reassurance that her problems are not uncommon, and education about symptoms to assist the client to obtain some type of control to help her adapt to the situation. A low-salt diet is encouraged and a diuretic (hydrochlorothiazide) may be ordered to deal with water retention, along with vitamin $B_6$ (50–100 mg/day) and vitamins A and E for breast symptoms.

16. **(4)** The vagina naturally cleanses itself, and therefore douching is not necessary unless prescribed by a health care provider to treat a medical condition. Douching should be avoided during menses to prevent infection.

## Gynecologic Disorders

17. **(1)** The initial outbreak is usually the worst. Herpes simplex type 2 can be transmitted even when there is no lesion present, and it cannot be cured. Vaginal delivery is allowed, if there are no genital lesions at the time of labor.

18. **(1)** Bacterial vaginosis results when the normal environment in the vagina is disrupted. The normal vaginal lactobacilli are decreased or absent, and there is an overgrowth of many different types of anaerobic bacteria. Trichomoniasis is caused by a flagellated protozoan, and gonorrhea is caused by a bacteria and may be asymptomatic. The virus that causes recurrent outbreaks of genital lesions is herpes genitalis type 2.

19. **(1)** OCs will reduce the production of prostaglandin, which is thought to be the primary cause of dysmenorrhea.

20. **(4)** The criteria for the diagnosis of bacterial vaginosis are characteristic milky homogeneous discharge, ph > 4.5, amine odor (positive whiff) with addition of potassium hydroxide (KOH), and the presence of epithelial cells studded with coccibacilli, which obscure the borders (clue cells). Pseudohyphae are present in candidiasis.

21. **(3)** Ninety percent of dysfunctional uterine bleeding is caused by anovulation. The lack of progesterone allows asynchronous, excessive proliferation of the endometrium. This tissue is fragile, and the normal hemostatic mechanism is altered. Thyroid disease, blood dyscrasias, and uterine tumors can mimic dysfunctional uterine bleeding and must be excluded.

22. **(3)** A female-appearing person with 46,XY karyotype is referred to as having androgen insensitivity syndrome, or testicular feminization. This maternal X-linked recessive disorder accounts for approximately 10% of all cases of amenorrhea, and these individuals appear normal until puberty. These clients then present with amenorrhea, scant or absent pubic hair, and abnormal or no breast development. Persons with Müllerian abnormalities have normal XX karyotype with abnormalities of fallopian tubes, uterus, and upper vagina occurring in fetal development. In Turner's syndrome, there is congenital absence of ovaries due to loss of one X chromosome.

23. **(1)** The most common breast mass in young women less than 30 years old is the fibroadenoma. This benign breast mass is the third most common breast mass after fibrocystic changes and carcinoma. Fibrocystic breast changes are seen most commonly in women 30–50 years old. Intraductal papilloma is a wart-like growth located in the mammary duct and occurs in women 40–50 years old. Malignant breast neoplasms occur most frequently in women over 40 and are rarely seen in women 15–25 years old.

24. **(1)** Nonsteroidal anti-inflammatory analgesics inhibit prostaglandin synthesis and are effective agents in primary dysmenorrhea. The other agents listed have not demonstrated effectiveness in primary dysmenorrhea. Other measures to decrease discomfort are exercise, relaxation techniques, heat application, and low-dose OCs.

25. **(4)** Secondary amenorrhea is defined as no menses for three cycle lengths or 6 months in a woman with previously established menses. Exercise can cause an increase in estrogen and endorphin levels, which influence the release of gonadotropin-releasing hormone (GnRH). Without appropriate GnRH release, FSH and LH are not released appropriately, resulting in anovulation, which may lead to amenorrhea. The other conditions listed are causes of primary amenorrhea.

26. **(1)** This has the characteristics of a syphilitic lesion and needs to be evaluated. Only after determining the presence or type of STD can it be treated effectively. The herpes viral culture should be done while the lesion is present and the fluid from the vesicles can be obtained.

27. **(3)** Pregnancy is the most common cause of amenorrhea in young women. It is important to rule out pregnancy in a female client with a problem of amenorrhea, even if she is very athletic. Interviewing the client regarding her sexual practices is unreliable. The presence or absence of pregnancy should be determined prior to other diagnostic studies.

28. **(2)** A person who has never engaged in coital activity is not considered to be at risk for cervical cancer, due to the unlikelihood of exposure to HPV. In addition to others not listed here, the presence of HPV, multiple sexual partners, and/or previous HSIL are considered to be risk factors in the development of cervical cancer.

29. **(1)** The pseudohyphae and spores on the wet mount (KOH) are diagnostic for *Candida*. *Chlamydia trachomatic* is diagnosed by DFA (or by chlamydia culture). Gonorrhea is diagnosed by a cervical culture and bacterial vaginitis shows clue cells on the wet mount prep.

30. **(2)** Vaginal bleeding in prepubertal girls usually reflects a localized problem in the vagina or uterus including vulvovaginal infections, excoriation secondary to pruritus, foreign bodies, sexual abuse, trauma, tumor, or a history of DES exposure (even though it is extremely unlikely that today's young females will have been exposed to DES in utero). Options #1, #3, and #4 are considerations for the pubertal girl.

31. **(3)** Herpes simplex virus type 2 commonly presents dramatically in the newly infected primary outbreak. Gonorrhea generally is associated with a mucopurulent vaginal discharge, and is not accompanied by vesicular lesions. Chlamydia can be associated with dysuria and, unless accompanied by pelvic inflammatory disease (PID), is not generally accompanied by fever or body aches, nor is it associated with vesicular lesions. Lymphogranuloma venereum is a rare disease classically accompanied by pustular enlargement of the lymph nodes, particularly the inguinal nodes. It is not associated with vesicles, but rather bubos.

32. **(2)** Screening lab blood work for glucose, CBC with differential, and TSH in this age group without any stated risk factors is not cost effective and is of little value. This client can be better served with a discussion regarding diet and exercise. Since this client is at risk for STDs, counseling and testing for these is a reasonable approach. Contraceptive information educates the client and allows her to make wiser choices in her family planning.

33. **(1)** The recommended age for a female to begin screening Pap smears is at the onset of sexual activity or at 18 years. Since this client is 19 years old and has not had her first Pap smear yet, this would be the most appropriate test to perform. It is not necessary to perform STD screening on clients who have not been sexually active. Stool hemoccult testing and mammography are not recommended as screening procedures in the young adult.

34. **(3)** The presence of bruising, particularly on genitalia, should raise the suspicion of abuse. Combined with her nonverbal behavior, the bruising should prompt the nurse practitioner to explore the possibility of abuse.

35. **(1)** Reactive cellular changes are most commonly associated with inflammation, including typical repair. Other causes include atrophy with inflammation (atrophic vaginitis), intrauterine device (IUD) use, radiation, and diethylstilbestrol (DES)-exposed daughters. OCs do not cause reactive changes, and estrogen vaginal cream may be used to improve atrophy.

36. **(2)** The exact cause of cervical disease is unknown. Evidence is increasing that sexually transmitted agents act as carcinogens. Viral exposure to herpes genitalis, HPV, and HIV is therefore considered a risk factor. Other risk factors are related to sexual activity, such as sex prior to 18 years of age, first pregnancy prior to 18 years of age, multiple sexual partners, high parity, and partners with carcinoma in situ of the penis.

37. **(2)** Symptoms are most likely indicative of benign fibroadenoma. Mammography is indicated. Surgical excision is unlikely for a young woman.

38. **(2)** Toxic shock syndrome occurs primarily in menstruating women ages 12–24 who use tampons. The diagnosis is made with the presence of fever over 102°F, macular rash, hypotension, and involvement of three or more organ systems.

39. **(4)** Almost half of all vaginal infections are due to candidiasis. The majority of women who develop the disease have recently taken antibiotics. It is not a STD or due to poor hygiene.

40. **(1)** It is important to evaluate the client for threatened abortion as soon as possible. It is most likely too soon for the CBC to reflect blood loss. A pelvic sonogram will take longer than a urine pregnancy test, and it is imperative that the client be immediately referred for a dilatation and curettage (D&C), if her pregnancy test is positive.

# Pharmacology

41. **(3)** Rocephin is a very effective drug for complicated urinary tract infection, but is unnecessary in the uncomplicated lower urinary tract infection. Bactrim DS and Macrobid are both very effective for treatment of urinary tract infection. Pyridium will help to make the client more comfortable until the antibiotic reaches effective levels for treatment.

42. **(3)** Fluconazole is now approved for single-dose oral treatment of uncomplicated vulvovaginal candidiasis. It is most

convenient for this client, who is unlikely to be extremely compliant with vaginal creams. She does not have any contraindications to its use. Metronidazole and clindamycin are treatments for bacterial vaginosis and not for *Candida* infections. Hydrocortisone is a topical steroid used for inflammatory dermatologic conditions, and, while it may help the itching, it would not treat the candidiasis.

43. **(4)** Metronidazole vaginal cream is the treatment of choice for bacterial vaginosis. The newest recommendations allow for its use once daily for 5 days. The use of doxycycline listed here is for treatment of uncomplicated vaginal *Chlamydia trachomatis*. Terconazole vaginal cream is used for vaginal candidiasis; acyclovir is used for treatment of Herpes simplex infections.

44. **(4)** Benzathine penicillin 2.4 million units IM is the treatment of choice for syphilis, but this client has condyloma acuminatum, not lata. Topical podophyllin or trichloroacetic acid and cryotherapy are all accepted treatment modalities for condyloma acuminatum.

45. **(3)** Metronidazole (Flagyl) in a single 2-gm dose is the treatment of choice for trichomoniasis. An alternative is dividing the 2 gm into divided doses given the same day. This regimen has less nausea and may improve compliance.

46. **(4)** Metronidazole (Flagyl) is the treatment of choice for bacterial vaginosis. However, pregnancy should be ruled out prior to beginning treatment because metronidazole should not be used if there is any possibility the woman is pregnant. The sexual partners do not have to be treated, and doxycycline is not the drug of choice.

47. **(3)** She requires added protection through this cycle because of the low-dose OC. Dilantin may also decrease the effectiveness of OCs, especially low dose.

48. **(3)** The most common cause of pelvic inflammatory disease in sexually active women is gonococcal infections. Gonococcal infections are often accompanied by chlamydia, and they are usually both treated.

# Mental Health

## Psychosocial Examination & Diagnostic Tests

1. The mental status examination enables the nurse practitioner to identify:

   1. Intelligence quotient and reasoning.

   2. Abstract thinking and memory functioning.

   3. Reasoning and psychomotor skills.

   4. Memory functioning and intelligence quotient.

2. An adolescent with a history of psychiatric problems arrives at the clinic shouting that he is a messenger of God and knows the meaning of the prophecies in Revelations. This behavior is assessed as:

   1. A delusion.

   2. A hallucination.

   3. Magical thinking.

   4. An illusion.

3. An assessment of an adolescent experiencing auditory hallucinations would most likely reveal:

   1. Adolescent mumbling to self, tilted head, eyes darting back and forth.

   2. Performance of obsessive–compulsive rituals of turning off and on a radio, talking to self.

   3. Hyperactivity, expansive mood, easy distractibility.

   4. Cool, aloof, unapproachable, avoiding enclosed areas.

4. The MAST and the CAGE are a screening instruments for which disease process?

   1. Glaucoma.

   2. Depression.

   3. Alcoholism.

   4. Diabetes.

5. When receiving the records from another agency, the nurse practitioner notes on the summary sheet that the client has a dual diagnosis. This means the client has:

    1. Both manic and depressive symptoms of bipolar affective disorder.

    2. Two closely related psychiatric disorders (e.g., panic disorder and bulimia nervosa).

    3. Coexistence of both a psychiatric disorder (e.g., depression) and a substance abuse disorder (e.g., alcohol dependence).

    4. Coexistence of a personality disorder (e.g., borderline personality) and a psychiatric disorder (e.g., panic disorder).

6. A child is being evaluated for attention deficit hyperactivity disorder (ADHD). Which test is helpful in evaluating the difference between ADHD and a learning disability?

    1. Standardized IQ achievement test.

    2. Denver developmental screening test.

    3. Audiologic and visual testing.

    4. Complete neurologic examination.

7. In taking a history from an adolescent with depressive symptoms, which is the most important question for the nurse practitioner to ask?

    1. Have you ever experienced hallucinations, delusions, or illusions?

    2. Have you ever been hospitalized in a psychiatric facility?

    3. Do you regularly take antidepressants or other medications?

    4. Have you thought about or attempted suicide?

8. While taking a history, the nurse practitioner is aware that which of the following drugs is most commonly used first by an adolescent?

    1. Nicotine. *Gateway drug*

    2. Alcohol.

    3. Marijuana.

    4. Crystal methamphetamine.

9. A common laboratory finding associated with bulimia nervosa is:

    1. Hyperkalemia.

    2. Hypochloremia.

    3. Elevated liver enzymes.

    4. Platelet abnormalities.

10. The nurse practitioner knows tolerance is suggested when a client gives a history of:

    1. The same dose of the drug having reduced effects.

    2. Less of the medication producing the desired effects.

    3. No withdrawal symptoms when the drug is stopped.

    4. Increasing side effects with an increase in the dosage of drug.

# Psychiatric Disorders

11. An adolescent calls the clinic and asks to speak to the nurse practitioner. When she answers the telephone, the adolescent states that he is going to commit suicide. The priority goal is to:

    1. Refer the adolescent to an appropriate treatment facility.

    2. Encourage ventilation of angry and depressed feelings.

    3. Assess the lethality of the suicide plan.

    4. Establish rapport with the adolescent.

12. During an intake interview with a 19-year-old diagnosed with generalized anxiety disorder, the nurse practitioner might observe what type of behaviors?

    1. An inflated sense of self.

    2. Constant relation to future events.

    3. Inability to concentrate and irritability when questioned.

    4. Nervousness and fear of the nurse during the interview.

13. While talking with an adolescent about his chemical dependency, the client states, "I wish I would have never used cocaine. It's ruined my life!" What would be the most appropriate response by the nurse practitioner?

    1. "You should think before you do something."

    2. "Things will work out, don't worry."

    3. "It sounds like you've thought a lot about your cocaine use."

    4. "You shouldn't be so hard on yourself. You can change."

14. The nurse would expect which symptoms in a client with a diagnosis of schizophrenia?

    1. High energy with varying sleep patterns and nonstop conversation.

    2. Extreme and frequent mood swings with hyperactivity and difficulty concentrating.

    3. Paranoia, delusions, hallucinations, and diminished self-care.

    4. Antisocial behavior, manipulativeness, charisma, and ability to lie convincingly.

15. A 16-year-old female, who recently got married to a man (10 years older than herself who plays the guitar in a rock band) to "get out of the house," presents to your clinic for the third time in 2 months with a complaint of headache, gastrointestinal upset with abdominal pain, and difficulty sleeping. Past exams have been essentially negative. You suspect the the adolescent is depressed but she has been reluctant to complete even the briefest of screenings for this. Today, she requests "something for sleep," again stating she "doesn't have time or the money to take a bunch of tests." Which diagnosis seems most likely?

    1. Hypochondriasis.

    2. Domestic violence.

    3. Addiction.

    4. Irritable bowel syndrome.

16. A 7-year-old child is diagnosed with a simple phobia to grasshoppers. The key symptoms include:

    1. Fear of being in a place where escape might not be possible.

    2. Avoidance of friends, complaints of stomach pains, and refusal to attend school.

    3. Fear of saying or doing something in public about grasshoppers that may be inappropriate or humiliating.

    4. Sweating, tachycardia, difficulty breathing, and light-headedness when a grasshopper jumps in front of his bicycle.

17. A mother brings her young child to the clinic, stating she fell off the porch swing. What assessment finding would cause the nurse practitioner to consider the possibility of child abuse?

    1. Mother is very upset and stroking her daughter's hair.

    2. Child is crying and says her head and arm hurt.

    3. Child has red-, blue-, and green-colored bruised areas on her trunk.

    4. Child has a bruised, edematous area on forehead and shoulder.

18. In evaluating a 16-year-old female client, which symptom would indicate anorexia nervosa?

    1. Refuses to discuss questions pertaining to food.

    2. Reflects a positive body image.

    3. States she is eating very well but has episodes of vomiting.

    4. The family states she refuses to stop her severe dieting.

19. A mother is concerned about her child having nightmares. The nurse practitioner understands that the difference between nightmares and night terrors is:

    1. Nightmares are vivid, frightening dreams recalled by the child.

    2. Nightmares rarely occur in children before age 4.

    3. Nightmares are accompanied by gross motor movements, labored breathing, and enuresis.

    4. Nightmares and night terrors are essentially the same and are unrelated to stressful events.

20. A 16-year-old adolescent is 54 inches in height. The nurse practitioner identifies the following as a positive effective coping behavior:

    1. Acts as the class clown.

    2. Has a rehearsed reply to teasing comments.

    3. Spends most of his free time watching television.

    4. Has predominantly friends who are short statured.

21. The nurse practitioner is examining an older adolescent who has been a long-term intravenous cocaine user. What other findings would alert to a frequent complication?

    1. Epistaxis and chronic rhinorrhea.

    2. Cardiac arrhythmias and hypertension.

    3. Chest congestion and wheezing.

    4. Hepatitis and cellulitis.

22. The nurse practitioner is comparing the typical signs of depression in the adolescent with those in the adult client. The depressed adolescent would present with:

    1. Lonely feelings.

    2. Sad, flat affect.

    3. Anger and acting-out behavior.

    4. Feelings of powerlessness and anxiety.

23. The effects of prenatal cocaine exposure on newborns include:

    1. Increased incidence of prematurity.

    2. Large for gestational age.

    3. Caput succedaneum.

    4. Hypotonia and lethargy.

24. While interviewing a teenager to determine her level of health, the nurse practitioner recognizes symptoms of anorexia nervosa. Which characteristic of anorexia nervosa would be noted in the initial assessment interview?

    1. Below to average intelligence.

    2. Increased libido.

    3. Vigorous daily exercise.

    4. Tachycardia.

25. The nurse practitioner expects a preschool child with ADHD to have:

    1. Delayed growth and development, especially language skills.

    2. Negativism, overactivity, and active curiosity.

    3. Diminished fine motor skills and frequent mood swings.

    4. Easy distractibility, impulsiveness, and fidgeting.

26. The nurse practitioner is completing a history and physical on a child who she suspects may be autistic. Findings associated with autism include:

    1. Delay in language development.

    2. Delay in physical growth.

    3. Overprotective parents who provide minimal social interaction for the child.

    4. Warm, cuddling child with excessive need for interaction.

27. The mother of a preschooler is concerned because her child has begun to stutter. The nurse practitioner should:

    1. Refer the child to a speech pathologist.

    2. Encourage the mother to correct the child when she stutters.

3. Give the child verbal exercises to perform at home.

4. Reassure the mother that stuttering is normal in a preschooler.

28. A teenage female client is brought to the nurse practitioner for evaluation by her grandmother with whom she lives. The teenager has been vomiting and her grandmother believes that she is becoming confused. The grandmother relates that the client has been upset lately over a breakup with her boyfriend. What will the nurse practitioner investigate as a possible cause for this teenager's symptoms?

1. Appendicitis.

2. Ectopic pregnancy.

3. Drug overdose.

4. Sexually transmitted disease.

29. A teenager comes to the office of the nurse practitioner and states that she was raped several hours ago by her boyfriend. The immediate action taken by the nurse practitioner is:

1. A pelvic examination to determine injuries to the client.

2. Assure her she will be examined by a trained provider who has a rape evidence collection kit.

3. Send her immediately for counseling to help her deal with this situation.

4. Call the client's parents so they can be with her.

30. Physical findings of cocaine abuse include:

1. Bradycardia, miosis, hypertension.

2. Hypertension, tachycardia, tremor.

3. Hypotension, bradycardia, abdominal cramps.

4. Decreased level of consciousness, tachycardia, excessive salivation.

31. While interviewing an adolescent female presenting with her mother for birth control counseling and examination, you detect signs of family tension. During the physical exam, while the mother is out of the room,

the daughter admits to frequent marijuana use and occasional drinking. Which of the following is included in an abuse assessment if you suspect family violence?

1. Signs of general neglect.

2. Injuries at different stages of healing.

3. Adolescent's response to a direct question.

4. Admitted fear of mother's boyfriend.

32. The parents of a 7-year-old boy ask advice regarding sugar intake, stating the child's teacher has said not to allow the child to have any sugar products such as cookies at lunch due to behavior problems. Advice would include:

1. The child needs further assessment for ADHD.

2. Moderate sugar consumption rarely produces inappropriate behavior.

3. Increase the protein and fat in his diet to decrease nerve overstimulation.

4. Research has shown increased sugar intake directly affects cognitive performance.

33. Which neurotransmitters are associated with the etiology of acute mania in bipolar affective disorder?

1. Epinephrine and norepinephrine.

2. Serotonin and dopamine.

3. Dopamine and norepinephrine.

4. γ-Aminobutyric acid (GABA) and renin-angiotensin.

34. All of the following behaviors meet the criteria of the *Diagnostic and Statistical Manual of Mental Disorders, Fourth Edition* (DSM-IV) for substance abuse, **except**:

1. Repeated arrests for drunk driving.

2. Multiple absences from work due to substance use.

3. Chronic anxiety attacks.

4. Recurrent arguments with spouse about his/her drinking behavior.

35. A mother brings her 14-year-old daughter to the clinic. She tells the nurse practitioner that she is concerned that her daughter is a lesbian. She relates that over the past couple of years she has noted that her daughter enjoys only masculine sports (i.e., football, baseball). The mother is concerned that her daughter wears her hair very short, refuses to wear dresses and makeup, dresses and acts like a "jock," and is not interested in dating or having female friends. The nurse practitioner understands that this is:

    1. Gender identity disorder.

    2. Lesbianism.

    3. Transsexualism.

    4. Cross-sex behavior.

# Pharmacology

36. What is a predominant side effect of methylphenidate (Ritalin) therapy for ADHD?

    1. Growth stimulation and delayed closure of epiphyseal plates.

    2. Hypertension and anorexia.

    3. Central nervous system (CNS) depression and rash.

    4. Bradycardia and dysrhythmias.

37. Which medication is a selective serotonin reuptake inhibitor (SSRI)?

    1. Amitryptyline (Elavil).

    2. Sertraline (Zoloft).

    3. Imipramine (Tofranil).

    4. Haloperiodol (Haldol).

38. The nurse practitioner understands that adolescents who use lysergic acid diethylamide (LSD) experience:

    1. Withdrawal symptoms within 24 hours.

    2. Quickly developing tolerance and need for increased amounts.

    3. Flashbacks and depression.

    4. Disorientation and delusional feelings.

39. In the management of acute alcohol withdrawal delirium, a nurse practitioner may want to use all of the following drugs **except**:

    1. Chlordiazepoxide (Librium).

    2. Lorazepam (Ativan).

    3. Thiamine.

    4. Chlorpromazine (Thorazine)

40. The nurse practitioner's physical exam of an adolescent is as follows: disheveled appearance, 5-lb weight loss since last visit 2 months ago, pulse strong and regular at 128, +4 deep tendon reflexes (DTRs), nasal mucosa erythematous, and ulcerated. His mother relates that he has been getting in trouble at school, avoids the family, has no appetite, and is not sleeping much at night. The nurse practitioner suspects use of:

    1. Heroin.

    2. Marijuana.

    3. LSD.

    4. Crack cocaine.

41. An adolescent comes to the rural clinic having taken an undetermined amount of heroin. Prior to transferring the adolescent to a psychiatric treatment facility, the nurse practitioner anticipates the drug of choice for an opioid overdose is:

    1. Clonidine (Catapres).

    2. Methadone (Dolophine).

    3. Naloxone (Narcan).

    4. Naltrexone HCl (Revia).

42. A school-age child is receiving methylphenidate (Ritalin). Which is an appropriate dosage schedule?

    1. 5 mg bid before breakfast and lunch; gradually increase dose to maximum of 60 mg/day.

    2. 20 mg qd in AM after breakfast.

    3. 1 mg tid before meals; gradually increase dose by 1 mg weekly to desired effect.

    4. 10–60 mg qd in two to three divided doses, preferably 30–45 minutes prior to meals.

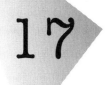

# Answers & Rationales

## Psychosocial Examination & Diagnostic Tests

1. **(2)** The mental status examination provides a basic assessment of the child's intellectual functioning (reasoning, abstract thinking, memory). The IQ is determined by psychological testing. Psychomotor skill assessment is part of a neurologic examination.

2. **(1)** Delusions are false, fixed beliefs that can be of a persecutory or grandiose nature. In this instance, the client is experiencing a delusion of grandeur. A hallucination is a false sensory experience. An illusion is a misinterpretation of reality. Magical thinking is when the client feels that his/her thoughts or wishes can control other people.

3. **(1)** Adolescents experiencing an auditory hallucination will often look out into space and act as if they are listening to someone talking. This is associated with behaviors such as tilting the head, mumbling, and eye movement.

4. **(3)** The Michigan Alcoholism Screening Test (MAST) and the CAGE (**C**ut down, **A**nnoyed, **G**uilty, **E**ye opener) are used to alert providers to the possibility of alcoholism.

5. **(3)** Dual diagnosis involves both a psychiatric diagnosis and a substance abuse diagnosis.

6. **(1)** Children with learning disabilities and ADHD are often impulsive, inattentive, and overactive. Usually, children with ADHD do not have lower IQ achievement scores; however, children with a learning disability usually demonstrate a level of educational achievement substantially below that of the IQ.

7. **(4)** Although the other questions are important to ask during the initial history, it is most important to ascertain whether or not the client has contemplated suicide. In addition, determination of a specific plan and the means to do it are also involved in the questioning about suicidal ideation.

8. **(1)** Nicotine is known as the "gateway drug" and is most commonly the first drug used by adolescents.

9. **(2)** The other abnormalities are not usually associated with bulimia. The hypochloremia is associated with the purging (self-induced vomiting).

10. **(1)** Tolerance exists when the same dose of the drug produces reduced effects; it is usually seen with the development of physical dependence.

# Psychiatric Disorders

11. **(4)** The nurse practitioner must first establish trust and rapport with the caller before an assessment can be made. If rapport is not established, the client will hang up the phone. The nurse practitioner understands that, by keeping the client talking, he is prevented from acting out the suicidal threat.

12. **(3)** Impaired concentration and irritability are major characteristics of generalized anxiety disorder. Clients are more focused on the here and now and have low self-esteem.

13. **(3)** The nurse's statement acknowledges the client's feelings and is open-ended, which promotes open discussion and helps the client clarify his feelings and thoughts. Option #1 is condescending and punitive. Option #2 offers false reassurance. Option #4 tends to discount the client's feelings.

14. **(3)** The characteristics of schizophrenia are delusions, tangential thought, suspiciousness, disorganized behavior, and hallucinations.

15. **(2)** The indicators of domestic violence in this case are the multiple vague physical complaints without supporting objective data, the suspected depression, and the reluctance to wait around in the clinic for extended periods of time. This adolescent is on the verge of disclosing, if a provider would only ask her about domestic violence.

16. **(4)** Simple phobias are characterized by symptoms of sweating, tachycardia, difficulty breathing, and light-headedness when coming in contact with the feared object. Option #1 describes true agoraphobia. Option #2 is often experienced with a child who has a school phobia. Option #3 refers to a social phobia.

17. **(3)** The nurse practitioner must determine whether the bruised areas match the type of trauma the parent describes. Bruises in various stages of healing turn different colors. Having different colored bruises indicates that the injuries have not occurred at the same time, which could be indicative of child abuse.

18. **(4)** Adolescents with anorexia nervosa will severely reduce their nutritional intake by dieting constantly on high fiber and low calories. They usually have an inappropriate body image.

19. **(1)** Nightmares peak in incidence around ages 3–4 years and are often associated with abandonment issues and posttraumatic stress disorder (following gun shootings, fires, abuse). Night terrors are typically accompanied by gross motor movements (sleep walking, enuresis), tachypnea, labored breathing, and tachycardia.

20. **(2)** Role playing and planning a rehearsed reply to teasing comments about short stature are helpful tools to deal with this issue. Although humor can be effective, constantly clowning around for attention is not positive coping behavior. Withdrawal (i.e., watching television or reading) is not effective coping and may indicate depression. Spending time and associating only with younger adolescents who are his height is not a positive coping behavior and may hinder normal maturation.

21. **(4)** More than 50% of intravenous cocaine users develop hepatitis, phlebitis, endocarditis, and acquired immunodeficiency syndrome. Epistaxis, rhinorrhea, and nasal congestion are seen most often in intranasal users of cocaine. Chest congestion, wheezing, and eventual emphysema occur in chronic free-base (crack) smokers. Although cardiac arrhythmias, hypertension, and respiratory arrest can occur, they are not the common complications.

22. **(3)** Adults who are depressed typically display findings noted in Options #1, #2, and #4. Adolescents often act out in defense, trying to protect themselves from feelings of vulnerability and dependency. Noting signs of anger and frustration in the adolescent is important to evaluate as the significance of the behavior may indicate symptoms of depression.

23. **(1)** The newborn exposed to cocaine is often premature and small for gestational age, has low birth weight, and has a low Apgar score. Intrauterine growth retardation occurs along with symptoms of hypertonia,

irritability, tremulousness, irregular sleeping patterns, and frequent gaze aversion.

24. **(3)** People with anorexia nervosa will exercise up to 4 hours a day. They are above average intelligence in most cases, suffer from bradycardia, and have decreased libido.

25. **(4)** In a preschool child, it may be difficult to distinguish ADHD as problems of overactivity, inattention, and negativism are common. Problems with language skill development along with fine motor skills are more likely found with learning disabilities. Active curiosity and negativism are normal behaviors for preschoolers.

26. **(1)** Autism is a developmental disorder that starts early in a child's life and is characterized by avoidance of eye contact, indifference to caregivers, language and communication delays, failure to develop a social smile, repetitive movements, and an excessive need for routine.

27. **(4)** Repetition of whole words and phrases is normal for preschoolers; therefore, it would be inappropriate to refer to a speech pathologist at this time. Parents should not correct or criticize the child. Verbal exercises are unnecessary and could be very stressful to the child.

28. **(3)** In teenage girls, the most common form of suicide attempt is by drug overdose. The combination of vomiting and confusion suggest a drug overdose.

29. **(2)** This client should be examined by emergency department personnel, many of whom are specially trained to collect the evidence needed to testify in court about the rape. The exam should not be done in the office unless the nurse practitioner has been trained in evidence collection and has a rape evidence collection kit. The exam must be done quickly before evidence is destroyed. The client decides who should be called for support. While she is encouraged to call her parents, she is also offered the support of a rape crisis center and other resources.

30. **(2)** Bradycardia and excessive salivation are not found with cocaine abuse. There are no drug antagonists that can be used for cocaine overdose, although naloxone is given to reduce the concurrent toxic effects of other narcotic drugs that may be in the client's body systems.

31. **(4)** While all of the answers may contribute to a nurse practitioner's suspicion of family violence, the admission of genuine fear of a household member is considered an excellent indicator of actual or potential violence and the level of danger in a home.

32. **(2)** Woraich's 1994 study failed to demonstrate a link between sugar and behavior or cognitive performance. Further assessment is indicated before labeling the child as having ADHD.

33. **(3)** Dopamine and norepinephrine (drugs that stimulate the noradrenergic and dopaminergic receptors) can precipitate mania or hypomania in clients. GABA and acetylcholine may also be neutrotransmitters involved in the process. In addition, stimulants such as amphetamines and cocaine can also cause manic-like symptoms.

34. **(3)** Chronic anxiety attacks are not part of the DSM-IV criteria.

35. **(4)** These are signs of cross-sex behavior in girls. It can be either a normal exploration of sex role behaviors (tomboy girls and sissy boys) or it can become a persistent, compulsive stereotyped pattern of gender identity disorder. Gender identity disorder is a rare condition and usually occurs before the onset of puberty, with cross-sex behavior patterns beginning before the age of 4.

# Pharmacology

36. **(2)** Classic side effects are due to CNS stimulation and include hypertension, anorexia, tachycardia, insomnia, dysrhythmias, blood dyscrasias, and rash.

37. **(2)** Zoloft has the shortest half-life of the currently marketed SSRIs. Elavil has the most anticholinergic and sedating side effects of the antidepressants and is classified as a tricyclic. Imipramine (Tofranil) is also a tricyclic antidepressant. Haldol is an antipsychotic medication.

38. **(3)** Flashbacks, depression, and psychotic behavior can occur with LSD use. There are no withdrawal symptoms or physical dependence associated with use. Commonly, the adolescent remains oriented but experiences hallucinations and altered bodily sensations.

39. **(4)** All of the drugs listed above may be used in acute alcohol withdrawal delirium, except chlorpromazine, which is an antipsychotic that has no use in the management of this condition.

40. **(4)** Often, some of the first indications of drug use in adolescents are related to a sudden change in behavior or school performance. Heroin use symptoms are constricted pupils, respiratory depression, needle tracks, and poor nutrition. Marijuana use symptoms are slow reflexes, tachycardia, conjunctival injection, nasal congestion, and increased appetite. LSD use symptoms are dilated pupils, reddened eyes, hypertension, increased appetite, and hallucinations. The use of CNS stimulants, such as crack cocaine, leads to hypertension, weight loss, anorexia, insomnia, hyperreflexia, and a perforated or ulcerated nasal septum.

41. **(3)** Naloxone is a narcotic antagonist and is used for the reversal of narcotic depression, including respiratory depression. Clonidine (Catapres) is a central $\alpha$-agonist and is indicated for treatment of hypertension. Methadone is used in the treatment of opioid addiction. The Food and Drug Administration (FDA) has placed methadone in a special drug category that allows medically supervised administration of the drug to addicts with chronic, intractable addictions to heroin. Naltrexone's therapeutic classification is narcotic detoxification adjunct.

42. **(1)** The correct dose schedule for children is 5 mg bid before breakfast and lunch, gradually increasing the dose to a maximum of 60 mg/day. The dosage schedule for adults being treated for narcolepsy is 10–60 mg qd in two to three divided doses, preferably 30–45 minutes prior to meals.

# 18 Emergencies

1. While attending a rural public school, a 7-year-old child was bitten on the hand by a raccoon. At the rural clinic, the nurse practitioner cleansed the wound. The next action is:

   1. Administer tetanus antitoxin.

   2. Contact local animal control authorities.

   3. Administer rabies immune globulin (RIG) and human diploid cell vaccine (HDCV).

   4. Teach the family how to do hourly soaks to the hand using normal saline and peroxide.

2. A toddler is brought to the clinic with a history of an insect bite last evening. What presenting symptom would be associated with the bite of a brown recluse spider?

   1. Paresthesias in all extremities.

   2. Edematous, erythematous area with coalescing macules.

   3. Tissue sloughing in the bite area within 8–10 hours.

   4. Development of a central black eschar or "sinking infarct" in 6–12 hours.

3. The nurse practitioner understands that cat bites become infected more often than dog bites because:

   1. Dogs have a "cleaner mouth" than cats.

   2. Cat bites are often deep puncture wounds.

   3. Dog bites are usually on the face, which makes them more susceptible to infection.

   4. Cat bites are usually associated with clawing and spreading of microorganisms.

4. When do most bites/stings from insects, spiders, snakes, and bees most commonly occur?

   1. Fall.

   2. Spring to fall.

   3. Winter.

   4. Any time of the year.

5. An adolescent was bitten on the face by a neighbor's dog 3 days ago. He has developed an infection in the wound area. What would be appropriate management of this client?

    1. Prescribe amoxicillin–clavulanate potassium (Augmentin) 250 mg PO tid × 14 days.

    2. Approximate the edges of the wound together with suture.

    3. Prescribe cephalexin (Keflex) 500 mg PO tid for 7 days.

    4. Have the adolescent return to the clinic for follow up in 2 weeks.

6. A young adolescent has been bitten by a black widow spider while doing yard work. He is having a severe reaction; the nurse practitioner expects:

    1. Hypotension and shock.

    2. Localized pain, erythema, and edema in the area.

    3. Black eschar of sloughing tissue within 4 hours of the bite.

    4. Abdominal rigidity, nausea, and headache.

7. A generally accepted acronym for snake bites is, "Red on yellow, kill a fellow; red on black, venom lack." A boy is bitten by a snake described as having broad rings of red and black separated by narrow rings of yellow. The nurse practitioner understands that the client experienced all **except**:

    1. Numbness and change in sensation.

    2. Local swelling at the fang mark site.

    3. Dizziness and diplopia.

    4. No symptoms, as the snake was not poisonous.

8. A father brings his 4-year-old son to the emergency room after the child ingested a small bottle of aspirin. The nurse practitioner's priority is:

    1. Insert a nasogastric (NG) tube and attach to low suction.

    2. Give 16 oz of orange juice.

    3. Give 8 oz of milk.

    4. Give 30 ml of syrup of ipecac followed by activated charcoal.

9. The nurse practitioner is aware that the toxic symptoms of salicylate poisoning are:

    1. Tinnitus and nausea.

    2. Itching and blurred vision.

    3. Fruity odor to the breath.

    4. Fever and chills.

10. The nurse practitioner understands that the most common cause of death in adolescents is:

    1. Acquired immunodeficiency syndrome.

    2. Motor vehicle accidents.

    3. Drug overdose.

    4. Congenital anomalies.

11. What is the most common cause of asphyxiation in childhood?

    1. Choking on food.

    2. Aspiration of a small object (i.e., marble, penny).

    3. Suffocation from head getting caught in the slats of an older crib.

    4. Suffocation by playing with a plastic bag or sleeping on plastic sheets.

12. Medical management for a brown recluse spider bite includes:

    1. Warm, moist soaks to the area.

    2. Ice pack and elevation of the area.

    3. Active and passive range of motion.

    4. Avoid use of antihistamines.

# 18  Answers & Rationales

1. **(3)** Any type of animal bite that might be associated with an animal that may potentially harbor rabies (skunks, bats, raccoons, foxes, coyotes, rats) should be treated with both active and passive rabies immunization. Tetanus antitoxin would be indicated if the child was not current on the immunization. Animal authorities would be called after the initial treatment to locate the animal and sacrifice it, so that the brain could be examined for rabies.

2. **(4)** Brown recluse spiders produce sharp pain at the instant of the bite, with subsequent minor swelling and erythema. Tissue necrosis may occur within 4 hours. A blue–gray to black macular halo may surround bite, with eventual widening and sinking of the center of the lesion, leading to a "sinking infarct" that leaves a deep ulcer that takes weeks or months to heal.

3. **(2)** Deep puncture wounds are more likely to get infected with anaerobic organisms. Bites on the hand have the highest infection rate, while bites on the face have the lowest infection rate.

4. **(2)** Insects are more active, reproduce, and are present in greater numbers in the warm months (i.e., spring to early fall).

5. **(1)** Amoxicillin–clavulanate potassium (Augmentin) is an excellent choice for the empiric treatment of animal bites. Keflex is not indicated due to resistant strains of *Pasturella multocida*, an organism present in 25% of dog bites and 50% of cat bites. An infected bite should be followed up on a daily basis, until the infection clears. Open wound management is indicated, not suturing.

6. **(4)** In addition to these symptoms, bronchospasm, hypertension, seizures, and altered mental status may occur. Black eschar is associated with a brown recluse spider bite.

7. **(4)** This was a poisonous coral snake bite. The typical symptoms are those listed plus the following: nausea, vomiting, and muscle fasciculations.

8. **(4)** An age-appropriate dose of syrup of ipecac followed by administration of activated charcoal would be indicated. The nurse practitioner would lavage the child, not insert an NG tube and attach to suction.

9. **(1)** Tinnitus and nausea are toxic symptoms of salicylate poisoning. Fruity odor to the breath is usually associated with diabetic ketoacidosis.

10. **(2)** Accidents and violence are the most common causes of death in the adolescent population.

11. **(1)** The most common cause is choking on food or fluids. Aspiration would probably be the second most common cause of asphyxiation. Suffocation is not the major problem due to more parent education about the problems associated with children playing or sleeping around plastic bags or materials.

12. **(2)** Heat application is contraindicated; ice packs are preferred, along with elevation to decrease the edema. The area should be immobilized. Tetanus toxoid may be given along with antihistamines to reduce swelling and relieve itching.

# 19

# Research & Theory

## Research

1. When designing a research project that will involve clients, from the options presented below, the most important point to be included in the written consent to participate is:

   1. The directions regarding the use of a black pen.

   2. The anticipated date for publication of the completed research report.

   3. The assurance of privacy and confidentiality.

   4. The number of previously published research studies about this topic.

2. When determining whether to incorporate a new procedure into your clinical practice based on the findings of a recent study, which of the following should you consider?

   1. The statistical significance of the findings.

   2. The statistical relevance of the findings.

   3. The statistical software program used.

   4. The statistical background of the researcher.

3. The research process is similar to the processes nurse practitioners use to provide client care in that both are decision-making processes that include the steps (in the order presented here) of:

   1. Assessing, teaching, evaluating, and discussing.

   2. Defining, planning, implementing, and charting.

   3. Questioning, evaluating, diagnosing, and teaching.

   4. Assessing, planning, implementing, and evaluating.

4. Both descriptive and inferential statistics are used in research. However, their purposes are different in that:

   1. Inferential statistics are used for assigning participant code numbers.

   2. Descriptive statistics are used for assigning participant code numbers.

   3. Inferential statistics are used for hypothesis testing.

   4. Descriptive statistics are used for hypothesis testing.

5. In an ambulatory care setting, the nurse practitioner might find it difficult to utilize nursing research because:

   1. The demands of providing primary care leave little time for research utilization.

   2. Procedures for research utilization have not been well defined in the literature.

   3. Research published in professional journals is too difficult to access by clinicians.

   4. Ambulatory care settings have little in common with the settings used for most research.

6. *Variance* is a key statistical concept. How would our current research methods change if there were no variance?

   1. We would need to increase the sample size in all of our research studies to 100 research subjects or greater.

   2. Since our current research methods do not depend on the presence of variance, we would not need to change our current methods.

   3. We would need to decrease the sample size of all our research studies to 15 research subjects.

   4. Since our current research methods are based on the presence of variance, we would not be able to use our current methods.

7. The scientific method for conducting research uses the null hypothesis, which is statistically based. The correct format for the null hypothesis is:

   1. There are no significant difference between two groups.

   2. Group "A" is greater than group "B."

   3. Group "A" is less than group "B."

   4. There is a 95% probability that group "A" is different from group "B."

8. When evaluating claims made on advertisements, such as "Drug X has been used for 5 years with over 1 million doses administered in the United States, Canada, and Great Britain. Drug X stops sinus congestion, and prevents cough for the

common cold, the nurse practitioner realizes that the claim is:

   1. Invalid as there is no control or comparison group and no statistics are stated.

   2. Valid as there are sufficient numbers of users who have had success.

   3. Invalid because the level of significance is not mentioned to be at the 0.05 level.

   4. Valid as the cohort and Hawthorne effect are operating.

9. In your practice, you have noticed that female clients who are pregnant and still in their early teens generally seem to go into labor before their due date (as determined by ultrasound), while the women who are in their late teens usually go into labor at or after their due date. Which statistical analysis would answer the research question, "Among pregnant women in a nurse practitioner practice, is there a statistically significant difference between the length of gestation for women ages 13–15 when compared to women ages 16–19?"

   1. Multiple regression.

   2. Chronbach's alpha.

   3. The two-tailed $t$-test.

   4. Pearson's correlation.

10. The utilization of research in nursing practice can be equated with:

   1. The nursing process.

   2. The change process.

   3. Discharge planning.

   4. Family planning.

11. You are compiling monthly statistics for your practice, and one of the elements of your analysis is the cultural background of your clients. What level of data is "cultural background"?

   1. Nominal level data.

   2. Ordinal level data.

3. Interval level data.

4. Ratio level data.

12. A nurse practitioner practicing with a physician in general practice is compiling the practice statistics at the end of the month. The clients who received care range from infants to the older adolescents. Of the following data from the monthly report, which is most likely to be normally distributed?

 1. The lab tests scheduled for the clients.

 2. The gender of the clients.

 3. The primary diagnosis of the clients.

 4. The age of the clients.

13. A nurse practitioner practicing with a physician in general practice is compiling the practice statistics at the end of the month. The nurse practitioner and the physician want to know the average monthly income of their clients. Which would be the most appropriate statistical measure of the "average income," assuming income was exact in dollars and cents?

 1. The mean.

 2. The median.

 3. The mode.

 4. The range.

14. A nurse practitioner is evaluating research articles for a utilization project. The majority of the articles report that either random selection or random assignment was used to select the sample for that study. Because certain procedures in research are used across disciplines, what can be assumed for studies where randomization has been used?

 1. The ages of the research subjects in these studies will be negatively skewed.

 2. The research subjects in these studies will automatically be half male and half female.

 3. The ages of the research subjects in these studies will be positively skewed.

 4. The researchers were attempting to obtain the most representative sample.

15. The ability to predict outcomes of care is desirable both in research and in practice. If a nurse practitioner wanted to create a theoretical model for a specific aspect of his/her practice to predict the client outcomes, which statistical analysis methods would be used to analyze the clinical data?

 1. Descriptive statistics.

 2. Repeated measures $t$-test.

 3. Multiple regression.

 4. Chi-square for independent samples.

16. Research articles are being evaluated for a utilization project. What can the nurse practitioner do if he/she does not understand the statistical procedures that were used for the analysis of data in an article?

 1. Assume that the correct procedure was used, and read about the method or consult a statistician for an explanation of the statistics.

 2. Assume that the article is beyond his/her ability to understand, so set that one aside and go on to the next article.

 3. Assume that the correct procedure was used and, instead of reading the results section, read the discussion of the findings section.

 4. Assume that the article is beyond his/her ability to understand and use someone else's critique of the reported study.

17. The nurse practitioner has determined that the office procedures for diagnosing and stabilizing new diabetics need to be evaluated and possibly changed. Which would be the best choice for the first phase of the evaluation?

 1. Design and conduct a double-blind clinical trial.

 2. Design and conduct a research utilization project.

 3. Design and conduct a research project comparing men and women.

 4. Design and conduct a study to test Callista Roy's theoretical model.

18. The nurse practitioner was reading a nursing research article in which there were no statistically significant findings. The most appropriate response would be:

    1. "Reading this article was a waste of my time."

    2. "Because of reading this article, there is no reason to conduct similar studies."

    3. "Reading this article raises new questions for my practice."

    4. "Because of reading this article, I will immediately change my practice."

19. The verification of the more abstract nursing theories (e.g., that of Martha Rogers) is often hampered by:

    1. The lack of adequate measures for the theoretical concepts.

    2. Prior studies that did not support the theory.

    3. The lack of adequate laboratory settings for conducting experiments.

    4. Prior studies that were conducted in other countries.

20. In a recently published study, the researcher reported "the statistical analysis used to identify the differences between the two variables was Pearson's correlation." Which most specifically tells what is wrong with this statement?

    1. Pearson's correlation can be used only with three or more variables.

    2. Pearson's correlation actually identifies the common factors between variables.

    3. Pearson's correlation can be used only when there is a single variable.

    4. Pearson's correlation actually identifies the relationship between variables.

21. Qualitative research studies are conducted by nurse researchers because:

    1. Qualitative studies help to identify and define nursing concepts.

    2. With qualitative methods, there are no concerns about the rights of research subjects.

    3. Qualitative approaches provide precise measures for statistical analysis.

    4. Nurse reachers find qualitative research designs easier to use.

22. The normal ranges of blood chemistry values are most like which statistical concept?

    1. The standard error.

    2. The mean.

    3. The standard deviation.

    4. The median.

23. The five major sequential steps of research utilization are:

    1. Establish a client relationship, perform a health assessment, make a diagnosis, devise a plan of care, evaluate the treatment.

    2. Identify the problem, assess published research, design the innovation, evaluate, decide whether to adopt the innovation.

    3. Review the popular literature, review the practice's clients, summarize the findings, evaluate, do client teaching.

    4. Review the client's lab reports, complete a thorough health assessment, diagnose, implément the treatment, evaluate.

24. Both *qualitative* and *quantitative* research methods are used in nursing research because:

    1. Master's-prepared nurses conduct quantitative studies, while doctorally prepared nurses conduct quantitative studies.

    2. Master's-prepared nurses conduct qualitative studies, while doctorally prepared nurses conduct quantitative studies.

    3. They compliment each other because they produce different types of findings about the same concepts.

    4. They compliment each other because they produce the same types of findings about different concepts.

25. Nursing research subscribes to the scientific method for the design of research studies. The advantage of this is that:

    1. Nursing research is based on logically constructed arguments.

    2. Nursing research is designed to answer any research question.

    3. Nursing research findings are precise and need not be duplicated.

    4. Nursing research findings are generalizable to all client populations.

26. With the restructuring of health care delivery and a shift in the provision of nonacute care from the hospital to ambulatory care settings and the home, previous nursing research that was conducted in hospitals:

    1. Now becomes applicable to all in-hospital providers of care.

    2. Remains relevant in the new settings; client care is unchanged.

    3. Should be applied directly to client care provided in the new settings.

    4. May no longer be applicable to the delivery of client care.

27. Nurse researchers strive to substantiate causality so that client outcomes can be consistently predicted. For the nurse practitioner, the ability to predict the outcomes for every client could mean that:

    1. The appropriate treatment would be prescribed for clients.

    2. No further studies would need to be conducted about treatments.

    3. The client's individual qualities would not need to be considered.

    4. Treatments would not need to be individualized for each client.

28. The reason that quantitative research articles always have a section containing descriptive findings is that descriptive data analysis:

    1. Provides the basis for making inferences about the findings.

    2. May yield statistically significant findings that were unexpected.

    3. Is conducted for predicting client outcomes in nursing settings.

    4. Organizes the data for clearer understanding of subjects and variables.

29. The difference between univariate and multivariate studies is:

    1. The number of subjects in the sample.

    2. The number of variables being studied.

    3. The number of sites for collecting data.

    4. The number of statistical hypotheses.

30. The theoretical basis for nursing practice is:

    1. A relatively new approach to nursing care.

    2. Borrowed from other professions such as medicine.

    3. As old as formal nursing and began with Florence Nightingale.

    4. Unrelated to the conduct of nursing research studies.

31. The independent variable and the dependent variable of a research study might be thought of as:

    1. The cause (the independent variable) and the effect (the dependent variable).

    2. The median (the independent variable) and the mode (the dependent variable).

    3. The outcome (the independent variable) and the treatment (the dependent variable).

    4. The sample (the independent variable) and the population (the dependent variable).

# Theory

32. While nursing theories vary greatly in their perspective of nursing care, all nursing theorists explicitly incorporate three key concepts. These three concepts, which are basic to nursing care, are:

    1. Individuals, families, and communities.

    2. Primary, secondary, and tertiary prevention.

    3. Past, present, and future well-being.

    4. Person, health, and environment.

33. Basing nursing practice on nursing theory contributes to the professionalization of nursing practice by:

    1. Adapting the medical model to nursing care.

    2. Limiting the choice of treatments for clients.

    3. Determining what type of clients will be seen by the nurse.

    4. Providing a consistent perspective for providing care to clients.

34. A nurse practitioner has decided to incorporate a nursing theoretical model into his/her practice. The practice includes clients of all ages. Which nursing model is most applicable to an ambulatory care setting?

    1. Orem's Model of Self-Care.

    2. Roy's Adaptation Model.

    3. Roger's Unitary Person Model.

    4. King's System Model.

35. Which nurse theorist is considered to have general systems theory as the philosophical orientation to her model?

    1. Sister Callista Roy.

    2. Martha Rogers.

    3. Rosemarie Parse.

    4. Betty Neuman.

36. Which nurse theorist addresses nursing outcomes in terms of primary, secondary, and tertiary prevention?

    1. Sister Callista Roy.

    2. Betty Neuman.

    3. Imogene King.

    4. Jean Watson.

37. Which nursing theorist's model primarily addresses health promotion?

    1. Jean Watson.

    2. Betty Neuman.

    3. N. J. Pender.

    4. Sister Callista Roy.

# 19 ▶ Answers & Rationales

## Research

1. **(3)** By federal law, clients must be assured of their privacy and confidentiality. The other information is interesting and may be included, but is not required by federal law.

2. **(1)** In published research reports, of the choices listed, only the first choice is consistently reported by researchers. The clinical relevance is considered, not the statistical relevance. The specific program used does not make a difference since all are based on the same statistical formulas. Researchers frequently work with statistical consultants so that a researcher's background is not a limitation to a published study.

3. **(4)** Only the last choice contains those elements common to both processes: assessing, planning, implementing, and evaluating.

4. **(3)** Only Option #3 is true. Neither is used to assign participant code numbers. Descriptive statistics are used to describe the sample.

5. **(1)** Inadequate time can be a barrier to research utilization in any setting. The process of research utilization is well delineated by researchers. With the ever-increasing availability of professional journals via the Internet, access is rarely a problem. There is a considerable body of research that has been conducted in ambulatory care settings.

6. **(4)** All our current research and statistical analysis methods rely on the presence of variance or variation; if variance is no longer present, our current methods could no longer be used. If there is no variance, a sample of 1 would be adequate.

7. **(1)** The correct format for the null hypothesis is "There are no significant differences between two groups." The alternate or research hypothesis may take the other forms.

8. **(1)** Even though the claims detail extensive use of Drug X, there must be statistical evidence as demonstrated through the use of control or comparison groups that will render a level of significance.

9. **(3)** Only the $t$-test compares two independent groups on a variable.

10. **(2)** Incorporating research findings into practice often results in a change in practice. The nursing process is most like conducting research.

11. **(1)** The variable of "cultural background" is categorical data or nominal-level data.

12. **(4)** The gender and primary diagnosis are nominal-level data, and the lab tests would be skewed, while the age would approximate the normal curve.

13. **(2)** The median income would be most representative of the average because the income of 50% of the clients is above and 50% is below the median. The mean could be influenced by one client with a very high or a very low income, and the mode only identifies the income that is reported most often. The range only identifies the lowest and the highest incomes and does not present an average.

14. **(4)** Randomization is a research technique used to increase the amount of control in any research design. The other three options are false; they do not occur because of randomization.

15. **(3)** Of the choices, only multiple regression examines the relationship between two or more variables in a way that permits prediction.

16. **(1)** In reviewing research, it is necessary to understand the statistical methods that the researcher used in order to determine the value of the study findings for the practice setting. The researcher's discussion may not provide the full extent of the findings, while someone else's critique may reflect a specific point of view that does not apply in very situation.

17. **(2)** As a first step, a research utilization project would provide a thorough review of the published literature on which to base a change. A full study may not be needed, and testing a theoretical model is not appropriate for this situation.

18. **(3)** The lack of significant findings is an important piece of information about the topic of the research, and definitely is not a waste of time. Particularly when findings are nonsignificant, more studies need to be conducted about this topic. Ideally, changes in practice are based on the findings of more than one study.

19. **(1)** The lack of adequate measures for theoretical concepts is a major roadblock in many areas of research, and particularly so with the more abstract theories. Prior studies always provide information about the theory, even when conducted in other countries. More abstract concepts tend not to be studied in lab settings.

20. **(4)** Correlations identify the relationships between variables. Two or more variables may be used. Factor analysis is used to identify common factors.

21. **(1)** The purpose of qualitative designs is to identify and define nursing concepts. Qualitative designs do not yield precise measures, are usually not analyzed statistically, are more difficult to use, and carry the same concerns about the rights of subjects as all other research designs.

22. **(3)** The normal ranges of blood chemistry values are based on studies that identified the standard deviation for each blood chemical. The mean and the median are averages, and the standard error is not applicable to this situation.

23. **(2)** This option contains the published steps. All other options are nursing actions taken on behalf of the client (in no particular order).

24. **(3)** The two methods do compliment each other because they produce different types of findings about the same concepts. The educational preparation of the researcher does not dictate the research method used.

25. **(1)** The scientific method is highly organized and is based on logical reasoning. Findings are rarely precise and studies do need to be duplicated. Some questions are not answerable by our current research methods. Because of small samples and other limitations, many findings from nursing research are **not** generalizable.

26. **(4)** Such a drastic change in health care delivery may make previous studies no longer applicable to nursing care. Health care restructuring has changed the way client care is provided.

27. **(1)** The ability to always predict client outcomes would mean that every client would receive the exact treatment for that individual. Treatments would still have to be individualized, and individual qualities would need to be considered. Because new treatments are always being devised, there would be a need for ongoing research.

28. **(4)** Descriptive data analysis does organize the data, and it facilitates understanding.

Descriptive statistics cannot be used for significance testing or for making inferences; inferential statistics are used. Predictions are made from studies that use inferential statistics.

29. **(2)** "Variate" refers to the number of variables in the study.

30. **(3)** The theoretical basis for nursing practice began with Florence Nightingale and has been used for practice and for research for over a century. Nursing theories are specifically developed for nursing.

31. **(1)** The independent variable may be considered the cause or the treatment, and the dependent variable may be considered the effect or the outcome. The median, mode, sample, and population are not designations for the independent or the dependent variables.

# Theory

32. **(4)** All current theories incorporate person, health, and environment. Other concepts may or may not be explicitly included in nursing theories.

33. **(4)** Theory-based practice contributes the consistent perspective that permits the comparison of care across settings. Theory-based practice does not necessarily limit treatments or determine client types. Theory-based practice specifically eliminates reliance on the medical model.

34. **(1)** Orem's theory focuses on the client participating and being in control of his/her own health care. Roy's model is most appropriate for acute care settings, Roger's for holistic health settings, and King's for a mental health setting.

35. **(4)** Betty Neuman's Health Care Systems Model, Imogene King's Systems Interaction Model, and Dorothy Johnson's Behavioral Systems are based on general systems theory. Roy's Adaptation Model is based on stress and adaptation as the framework. Martha Rogers' Science of Unitary Human Beings and Rosemarie Parse's Human Becoming Model are based on a humanistic developmental framework.

36. **(2)** Betty Neuman identified the need to implement nursing interventions through use of one or more of three prevention modalities (primary, secondary, and tertiary prevention).

37. **(3)** Pender's Health Promotion Model is an excellent nursing model that readily fits into a nurse practitioner's scope of practice. The other theorist's models are: Betty Neuman's Health Care Systems Model, Jean Watson's Human Science and Human Model of Caring, and Roy's Adaptation Model.

# Issues & Trends

1. Considering the four advanced practice roles of clinical nurse specialist, nurse practitioner, certified nurse midwife, and nurse anesthetist, which role became accepted by and included into the practice arena without significant controversy?

   1. Clinical nurse specialist.

   2. Nurse practitioner.

   3. Certified nurse midwife.

   4. Nurse anesthetist.

2. Historically, who was one of the most outspoken opponents of the nurse practitioner role?

   1. Loretta Ford.

   2. Hildegard Peplau.

   3. Martha Rogers.

   4. Dorothea Orem.

3. Who started the first nurse practitioner program?

   1. Hildegard Peplau.

   2. Mary Breckenridge.

   3. Agnes McGee.

   4. Loretta Ford.

4. Which is the most important aspect in developing health policy skills in the nurse practitioner?

   1. Develop political allies in Congress.

   2. Work on a campaign.

   3. Support causes such as teen pregnancy or acquired immunodeficiency syndrome.

   4. Write letters and editorials.

5. Which is the least important barrier to collaborative advanced nursing practice?

   1. Prescriptive authority.

   2. Reimbursement privileges.

   3. Legal scope of practice.

   4. Political activism.

6. For the nurse practitioner to obtain reimbursement, an understanding of which is important?

   1. Minimum Nursing Data Set (MNDS).

   2. ICD-9-CM, CPT, and HCPC codes.

   3. HCPC codes and NANDA diagnosis.

   4. Medicare and Medicaid number.

7. Steps of the change process according to Kurt Lewin are:

    1. Unsolving, mobilizing, recruiting, finalizing.

    2. Build relationships, acquire resources, choose solution, stabilize.

    3. Unfreezing, moving, refreezing.

    4. Forming, storming, norming.

8. What was the major impetus for nurse practitioner development?

    1. Need for an expert nurse clinician.

    2. Shortage of primary care physicians.

    3. Trend for specialized nurses to diagnose and manage unstable acute and chronic clients.

    4. Movement of graduate nursing education to diagnosis and treatment of major illness.

9. The nurse practitioner understands that Medicare B provides:

    1. Hospitalization costs for the insured.

    2. Health insurance benefits for low-income families.

    3. Benefits that cover physicians, nurse practitioners, medical equipment, and outpatient services.

    4. Outpatient laboratory and radiography services and skilled nursing care in appropriate facilities.

10. What is the impact of the Balanced Budget Act of 1997 on nurse practitioner practice?

    1. Authorizes all states to provide nurse practitioners prescriptive authority.

    2. Provides for only well visits and primary care services.

    3. Prevents a physician from billing 100% for a nurse practitioner's services.

    4. Allows direct Medicare payments to nurse practitioners in both rural and urban settings.

11. In the clinic, you have observed the following: one medical assistant is usually pleasant and helpful; the other is often abrasive and angry. The most important basic guideline to be observed by the nurse practitioner who must resolve a conflict between two medical assistants is:

    1. Require the medical assistants to reach a compromise.

    2. Weigh the consequences of each possible solution.

    3. Encourage ventilation of anger and use humor to minimize the conflict.

    4. Deal with issues, not personalities.

12. A male nurse practitioner approaches another nurse practitioner who is his friend and tells him that one of the female physicians at the clinic often follows him into the supplies room and tells him how good looking he is. Yesterday, she patted his hand and said, "I wish we would get to know each other better. I would make it worth your while—better benefits at the clinic, more money." The male staff nurse asks his friend, "What do I do? I don't want to date her, but I don't want to lose my job. I just want her to leave me alone!" The best reply for the friend would be:

    1. "Tell her that her behavior makes you feel uncomfortable and that you want her to stop."

    2. "Go for it!! Date her and see if you get what she promises."

    3. "Go ASAP to the human relations office at the agency and relate to them the entire situation."

    4. "Contact your lawyer and get advice ASAP, in case she decides to turn the tables and accuse you of advances."

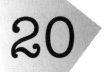

# Answers & Rationales

1. **(1)** According to the National Commission on Nursing (1983) and the Task Force on Nursing Practice in Hospitals (1983), the clinical nurse specialist (CNS) role was accepted quite rapidly. The psychiatric clinical nurse specialist role is considered the oldest and most highly developed of the CNS specialities and helped initiate the growth of other CNS specialities.

2. **(3)** Martha Rogers argued that the development of the nurse practitioner role was a ploy to lure nurses out of nursing and into medicine, hence weakening and undermining nursing's unique role in health care. This led to a major division within nursing, which led to barriers in the establishment of nurse practitioner educational programs within the mainstream of graduate nursing education.

3. **(4)** Loretta Ford, R.N., Ph.D., and Henry Silver, M.D. established the first pediatric nurse practitioner program at the University of Colorado. Mary Breckenridge established the Frontier Nursing Service in the depressed rural mountain area of Kentucky which led to training nurse midwives. Agnes McGee is credited with offering the first postgraduate program for the nurse anesthetist role at St. Vincent's Hospital in Portland, Oregon. Hildegard Peplau started the first psychiatric clinical nurse specialist program at Rutger's University.

4. **(1)** Although all of these answers are important for the nurse practitioner to develop policy skills, the most important is developing political allies. Having political allies in decision-making places (legislature) will enable the nurse practitioner to be active and informed regarding issues surrounding regulation, limitations on admitting privileges and prescriptive authority, and managed care.

5. **(4)** There are three major issues that are central to the expansion of the nurse practitioner role—prescriptive authority, reimbursement privileges, and legal scope of practice. Although political activism is important, it is not specific to collaborative practice.

6. **(2)** The ICD-9-CM (*International Classification of Disease, 9th Edition*) codes are diagnostic codes that identify the condition, illness, or injury to be treated and are used for billing insurance carriers. CPT codes (Physician's Current Procedural Terminology) specify the procedure or medical service given (over 7000 terms) Medicare and state Medicaid carriers are required by law to use CPT codes. The Health Care Financing Administration Common Procedure Coding System (HCPC) is used for reporting supplies and medical equipment.

7. **(3)** Lewin described three processes of change: unfreezing—involves breaking the habit, disturbing the equilibrium; moving—development of new responses based on new information with a change in attitudes, feelings, behaviors, or values; and refreezing—reaching a new status quo and stabilizing and integrating new behaviors with appropriate support that is available to maintain the change. Forming, storming, and norming refer to the stages of group process development. Option #2 is Havelock's change theory steps.

8. **(2)** According to most sources, the nurse practitioner role developed due to a shortage of primary care physicians in the 1960s and 1970s, when medical specialization was the trend.

9. **(3)** Medicare is regulated by the federal government and includes the services described, plus outpatient laboratory and radiography. Hospitalization costs are covered under Medicare Part A.

10. **(4)** A crucial and significant piece of legislation that allows direct payments to nurse practitioners at "80% of the lesser of either the actual charge or 85% of the fee schedule amount of the same service if provided by a physician." This does not change the "incident to" rule, which allows a physician to bill for 100% for a nurse practitioner's services, providing the physician is in the suite at the time of the service and readily available to provide assistance.

11. **(4)** Conflict must be addressed directly by the nurse practitioner. The personal characteristics of each of the medical assistants must not enter into the conflict resolution process. Determine what is the issue of conflict and then work on possible solutions to resolve the issue. Compromise is just one method of conflict resolution wherein both parties must be willing to give up something.

12. **(1)** There are two ways to deal with sexual harassment at work: informally and formally through a grievance procedure. Always start with the direct approach; ask the person to STOP! Tell the harasser in clear terms that the behavior makes you uncomfortable and that you want it to stop immediately.

# 21 Legal & Ethical Issues

1. An occurrence-form professional liability insurance policy is preferred because:

   1. The amount of insurance money available to pay a claim increases with each renewal of the policy.

   2. The policy proceeds are available to pay claims regardless of when the claim is reported to the carrier.

   3. The carrier will be notified of a potential claim during the policy period.

   4. The coverage is broader than that provided by a claims-made policy form.

2. Early reporting of a potential professional liability claim is advantageous because:

   1. Insurance carriers have a 10-day reporting window after which the coverage is canceled.

   2. Documents and witnesses needed to defend the claim are more likely to be available at the time of the event.

   3. Your insurance premiums will be reduced upon a good-faith showing of cooperation with the carrier.

   4. Risk Management personnel require such reporting in order to comply with Joint Commission on the Accreditation of Healthcare Organizations (JCAHO) mandates.

3. Your nursing license may be in jeopardy if:

   1. You appropriately delegate medication administration to a trusted registered nurse employee, who administers a fatal dose.

   2. You delegate client assessment tasks to a licensed practical nurse (LPN) who has been floated to your outpatient clinic for the day.

   3. You provide nursing care services consistent with established standards of practice in your jurisdiction.

   4. The medical assistant in your supervising physician's office exceeds the scope of her authority, but you take prompt action to correct the problem.

4. Your client is a 18-year-old adolescent woman with metastatic cancer. She has systematically secured enough pain medications to successfully end her life; she asks you to mix the drugs for her in some pudding to make them palatable for ingestion. Your best course of action would be:

1. Mix the medications as requested and stay with her while she consumes the preparation.

2. Consult with her parents and attending physician to warn them about the adolescent's proposed course of action.

3. Seek an immediate order for an antidepressant.

4. Sit down with the adolescent and her family and conduct a physical and psychological needs assessment.

5. The Patient Self-Determination Act (PSDA), passed by Congress in 1990, resulted in which of the following policy changes?

1. Hospitals are mandated to assist every client to create a "living will."

2. Federally-funded managed care organizations (MCOs) are required to inform subscribers about their rights under state law to create advance directives.

3. Home health agencies are required to have "do not resuscitate" orders on file for all terminally ill clients.

4. Hospitalized clients are obligated to select a surrogate decision maker to make health care decisions for them if they become incapacitated.

6. Both the Food and Drug Administration (FDA) and the Department of Health and Human Services (DHHS) have regulations governing research activities on human subjects. The principal investigator is responsible for:

1. Securing a signed special research consent form.

2. Reporting back to the Institutional Review Board if a subject is injured during the course of the study.

3. Appearing before the Institutional Review Board to present the study and secure approval to proceed with subject recruitment at the facility.

4. All of the above.

7. If you are served with a summons and complaint (i.e., lawsuit documents), the first step you should take is:

1. Call the client to determine the basis for the action and what you allegedly did wrong.

2. Call the client's lawyer (listed on the first page of the lawsuit) to get more information about the case.

3. Call your insurance company for instructions on how to proceed.

4. Confer with your colleagues and review the chart to see if you need to clarify your notes.

8. As a nurse practitioner in an impoverished rural area, you frequently encounter families in situations of domestic violence with few community options for referral. Participating in community education forums and fund-raising for a safe house is an example of applying the ethical principle of:

1. Autonomy.

2. Nonmaleficence.

3. Justice.

4. Veracity.

9. Nurses practicing in expanded roles should carry professional liability insurance for which of the following reasons?

1. Premiums are often modest and are a tax-deductible business expense.

2. Even if the employer insures the nurse practitioner, there may be situations of conflict between employer and nurse necessitating separate legal counsel, a covered benefit under the policy.

3. As roles expand, so does the liability potential.

4. All of the above.

10. The confidentiality of medical records is always a valid concern, especially in this age of computerization, "smart cards," and fax machines. Release of medical information to third parties is:

    1. Addressed mainly in state laws or statutes.

    2. Prohibited without the informed consent of the client.

    3. Automatic when the requesting party is a third-party payor or insurer.

    4. Disallowed if the records contain proof of a diagnosis of acquired immunodeficiency syndrome (AIDS).

11. Which categories of persons are **not** included in the definition of disability under the Americans with Disabilities Act (ADA)?

    1. Profoundly deaf employees.

    2. Persons who are wheelchair-bound.

    3. Current users of illegal drugs.

    4. Persons with mental retardation.

12. Bioethical practice dilemmas are best described as situations in which proposed treatment alternatives are:

    1. Ranked from most to least acceptable.

    2. Not appealing to involved parties.

    3. Lacking acceptance by anyone.

    4. Less than perfect approaches to the situation.

13. Health policy theorist Daniel Callahan believes that our health care system could be improved by:

    1. Making the care of the chronically ill our first priority, so that these individuals are not abandoned by the health care system.

    2. Making preventive care the first priority.

    3. Maintaining the current allocation of dollars to high-tech care.

    4. Leaving the system "as is" and letting market forces determine the allocation of health care dollars.

14. If a piece of equipment malfunctions while being used on a hospitalized child, the risk manager would probably recommend the following course of action:

    1. Return the item to the manufacturer with a description of the problem and a request for analysis.

    2. Tag and sequester the item at the facility and defer analysis pending risk management review of the litigation potential.

    3. Send the item to the biomedical engineering department with a request for immediate equipment breakdown and troubleshooting.

    4. Repair the item, either in-house or by an outside contracted firm, and return it to service ASAP.

15. Nurse expert witnesses are essential in the adjudication of most professional negligence claims against nurses. Which of the following criteria for nurse experts are sought by attorneys:

    1. Appropriate professional education, preferably at the technical level.

    2. Relevant and recent professional work experience.

    3. Ability to understand and articulate the legal issues involved in the claim.

    4. Published authors of medical texts in the clinical subject areas.

16. Which federal law mandates the tracking of implantable medical devices?

    1. The Administrative Procedures Act (APA).

    2. The Patient Self-Determination Act (PSDA).

    3. The Safe Medical Devices Act (SMDA).

    4. The Omnibus Budget Reconciliation Act (OBRA) of 1987.

17. Which of the following are elements of a broad-based risk management program?

    1. A hazardous materials compliance program as part of a comprehensive safety and security system.

    2. An early-warning/incident reporting program to identify elements of risk.

    3. A system of contract review to avoid assuming liabilities that should be borne by others.

    4. All of the above.

18. The type of insurance coverage that is purchased (or self-insured) by an organization to handle employee job-related injuries is:

    1. Professional liability insurance.

    2. Business interruption insurance.

    3. Directors and officers insurance.

    4. Workers' compensation insurance.

19. While driving your personal vehicle on a job-related errand, you are struck by a semi on the interstate. The car is totaled and you are severely injured. Which insurance policies will respond to these losses?

    1. Your personal auto policy and your employer's workers' compensation policy.

    2. The employer's business auto policy and workers' compensation.

    3. Your homeowner's policy.

    4. The semi driver's personal auto policy.

20. Nurse practitioners with hospital privileges may be impacted by the part of the Health Care Quality Improvement Act known as the National Practitioner Data Bank. Which of the following statements about the Data Bank is **not** true?

    1. Professional liability insurance claims payments made on behalf of nurse practitioners must be reported to the Data Bank.

    2. The facility granting medical staff privileges must query the Data Bank before approving a practitioner's privileges.

3. The purpose of the Data Bank is to have a national source of information about malpractice claims, licensure action, and restrictions on privileges so that practitioners may not easily move from one jurisdiction to another to escape quality review.

4. Insurance companies report all malpractice payments made on behalf of affected practitioners, regardless of the amount of the payment.

21. In 1985 Congress took action against a phenomenon known as "patient dumping" by enacting what was known at the time as the COBRA law, now referred to as the Emergency Medical Treatment and Active Labor Act (EMTALA). Which statement about EMTALA is **not true**?

    1. The original purpose of the statute was to prohibit the transfer of uninsured and untreated clients from the emergency department of one hospital to another (usually the county hospital).

    2. Subsequent rules and case law have expanded the statute so that almost any unauthorized transfer of a client from one facility to another is potentially problematic.

    3. In order to effect a proper transfer, the forwarding facility need not notify or secure the acquiescence of the receiving facility.

    4. The transferring facility must utilize appropriate transport methods and send copies of clients' medical records.

22. You are a nurse practitioner wishing to effect change in the state's laws regarding the dispensing of prescription medications by nurse practitioners. You would take your case to:

    1. The state legislature.

    2. The state board of nursing.

    3. The state board of pharmacy.

    4. The nursing specialty organization.

23. The common meaning of "gag clauses" or "gag orders" in the managed care arena is:

1. The MCO declines to publish, in its subscriber contracts, the treatments that are excluded from coverage under the plan.

2. The MCO refuses to allow its member services personnel to answer certain subscriber questions about covered benefits.

3. MCO contracts with providers disallow providers' offering treatment alternatives that the providers know are not covered by clients' plans.

4. Providers are prohibited from offering experimental treatment to clients.

24. Under the Safe Medical Devices Act of 1990, the following health care providers or organizations are required to report the death of a client to the FDA if the death is related to the use of a medical device:

1. Physicians' office staff.

2. Hospitals, home health agencies, and ambulance companies.

3. Nurse family members treating clients without compensation.

4. Physicians making home visits.

25. A young client receives a medication that was intended for another person. An appropriate way to document this event in the medical record would be:

1. "Client was given $x$ mg of $y$ drug in error."

2. "$x$ mg of $y$ drug administered to client. No adverse effects noted. Physician notified."

3. "Client received wrong medication. Incident report filed. Practitioner disciplined."

4. "Practitioner inadvertently administered $y$ drug to wrong client. Supervisor notified. Family threatening litigation."

26. The one reason that clients offer, above all others, for suing practitioners for medical negligence is:

1. The care they received was substandard.

2. The provider made an honest mistake.

3. The client wasn't "heard" when he/she attempted to communicate with the provider.

4. The client participated fully in all aspects of medical decision making, but the results were disappointing.

27. Informed consent is based upon the ethical principle of:

1. Beneficence.

2. Respect for persons.

3. Nonmaleficence.

4. Autonomy.

28. The four elements of a professional negligence claim are:

1. Duty, fulfillment of duty, professional relationship, and wrongful act.

2. Professional responsibility, fault, harm to the client, and wrongful act.

3. Duty, breach of duty, causal connection between the act and the harm, and harm to the client.

4. Professional relationship, intentional wrongful act, proximate cause, and damage to the client.

29. An expert witness is usually required in a nursing negligence case because:

1. Knowledge of medical or nursing facts is not considered intuitive to a lay jury.

2. Jurors are allowed to use their "sixth sense" regarding the facts presented to them.

3. Fact witnesses are not able to present an unbiased account of the circumstances in dispute.

4. Appropriately credentialed experts have more credibility in the eyes of lay jurors.

30. The standard of care for a nurse practitioner, in a trial, will be established by expert witness(es). The expert opinion will be based upon:

1. National norms for the specialty.

2. Facility policies and procedures.

3. Professional literature.

4. All of the above.

31. Alternative Dispute Resolution (ADR) is a process wherein the parties to a dispute resolve their differences outside of a court trial. Advantages to this system of problem solving include all **except**:

    1. The parties usually prefer the process because they have their opportunity to be heard in a less formal and less intimidating environment.

    2. The process is often less time-consuming and less costly than traditional litigation.

    3. Damage awards are less likely to include nonfinancial compensation.

    4. Insurers are amenable to working with mediators with a track record of fairness and successful case resolution.

32. The statute of limitations is:

    1. The state law that prescribes the time frames within which a nursing negligence action may be filed.

    2. The law that states that minors have no legal authority to sue nurses for malpractice.

    3. The law that limits the right of clients to sue nurse practitioners for negligent acts.

    4. The federal law that limits a nurse practitioner's right to countersue a client for malicious prosecution.

33. You are a nurse practitioner driving along the interstate on your way to a nursing seminar. You observe a head-on collision and decide to stop to render aid. Which statement is **false** with respect to your potential liability for malpractice?

    1. You had no legal obligation to stop to render assistance; if you had driven by the accident, there would be no liability on your part.

    2. If you provide appropriate nursing care, gratuitously, you will be protected from liability under your state's Good Samaritan Law.

    3. Even if you act in a grossly negligent manner, the Good Samaritan Law will shield you from liability.

    4. The protections afforded by the Good Samaritan Law may differ from state to state; you should research your state's law on the subject.

34. If you are subpoenaed to appear for a deposition in a nursing negligence case, appropriate preparation is prudent. One of the following tips would probably not be suggested by your attorney. Which piece of advice is **not** appropriate?

    1. Discreetly chew gum to calm your nerves, and dress for dinner because depositions usually take all day and you will not have time to change.

    2. Review the client's medical record and any other materials suggested by your attorney prior to your appearance for questioning.

    3. Take as much time as you need to think about your response before answering; do not let an attorney put words in your mouth.

    4. Be straightforward and truthful; remember that "I don't know" and "I don't remember" are acceptable responses.

35. Which of the following documentation tips is **not** a good idea?

    1. Carefully document your criticism of a fellow provider's clinical decision in the client's medical record. This will protect you if your treatment decisions needs to be defended later.

    2. Use standard abbreviations in the medical record so that subsequent readers will have no doubt as to your meaning and intent.

    3. Document telephone conversations with the client and/or the family in the medical record. Be particularly vigilant about recording changes in the client's medications.

    4. Document noncompliant client behaviors in the medical record; be thorough, yet factual.

36. If a client is under the age of majority in your state, what factors would you consider in order to determine if the client is "emancipated" and able to consent to medical treatment?

1. Whether the client is married.

2. Whether the client is in the military.

3. Whether the client is living outside the "care, custody and control" of a parent or guardian.

4. All of the above.

37. In 1987, and again in 1994, Congress acted to update many of the regulations that govern the provision of long-term care services. If you are an employer or nurse manager in this environment, you need to know that:

    1. Nursing assistants working in long-term care facilities must be formally trained and certified.

    2. Clients or residents have specific rights, such as information about their physical condition, medical benefits, and associated costs.

    3. New and swifter sanctions are available to reviewers to impose upon facilities with deficiencies.

    4. All of the above.

38. You are employed as a nurse practitioner in a private medical office. You notice all the activity at the front desk, where some families are checking in for appointments, staff is scheduling tests, and telephone advice triage is in progress. To preserve client confidentiality, you could implement which of the following changes?

    1. Orient the fax machine and computer monitor such that incoming reports or other data cannot be read by non–staff members.

    2. Do all telephone scheduling from a more secure location, such as a conference room in the back office.

    3. Create a more private space to confer with families who need follow-up information or explanations of tests or treatments.

    4. All of the above.

39. As a nurse-employer, you would be well advised to have procedures in place to appropriately terminate an employee. To avoid a charge of discrimination or a claim

of wrongful termination, you should be particularly sensitive to the protections afforded to select groups. Which of the following is **not** a protected class under the antidiscrimination statutes?

1. Pregnant women.

2. Gay men.

3. Those age 40 and older.

4. The handicapped.

40. Which activity could be considered grounds for a sexual harassment claim?

    1. A male employee tells an off-color joke to another man. The joke is overheard by a female co-worker who seems to appreciate the humor in it. The joke-telling is an isolated incident.

    2. A nurse-supervisor conducts an employee performance review. The supervisor does not mention a prior social relationship with the employee; the ratings are appropriate for the level of performance; the employee receives a salary increase.

    3. A co-ed locker room is decorated with multiple centerfold photos from a popular men's magazine. The female employees find this offensive and have filed several complaints.

    4. A nurse is complimented on her appearance and asked on a date by her boss. She informs the boss that she is married and not seeking another relationship. The incident is forgotten.

41. The purpose of the Americans with Disabilities Act (ADA) is:

    1. To level the playing field with respect to employment and other opportunities for disabled people.

    2. To create a federal entitlement program for people with AIDS.

    3. To guarantee wheelchair access to every residential and commercial building.

    4. To authorize interpreters for deaf employees at all private businesses.

42. As a result of the U.S. Supreme Court's ruling on assisted suicide, the current state of the law on this topic is:

    1. Assisted suicide is still a criminal offense in most jurisdictions.

    2. A physician may prescribe a fatal dose of medication with the concurrence of the ethics committee.

    3. A nurse practitioner may prescribe a fatal dose of medication with the concurrence of the supervising physician.

    4. A pharmacist may instruct a client how to mix and ingest a fatal dose of prescription medication.

43. A professional negligence or medical malpractice case is a civil action. The difference between a civil lawsuit and a criminal lawsuit is:

    1. The damages sought in a civil suit are monetary; one private party sues another for money.

    2. If you are convicted in a criminal case, you are still covered by your professional liability insurer.

    3. In a criminal case, your state sues you for money; other penalties do not apply.

    4. In a civil suit, if you do not prevail you could be incarcerated.

44. Which of the following is **not** a form of alternative dispute resolution (ADR)?

    1. Mediation.

    2. Binding and nonbinding arbitration.

    3. Settlement conference.

    4. A jury trial.

45. It is particularly important for nurses who care for children to have adequate professional liability insurance coverage because:

    1. Damages are always higher when a child is the injured party.

    2. Juries tend to award fewer dollars to injured children because the children are eligible for a variety of social programs that cover their medical expenses.

    3. The statute of limitations is often tolled (put on hold) until the minor reaches majority, so the time frame within which the child can file a lawsuit is extended.

    4. Insurers are sensitive to the increased risk posed by minor claimants, so the coverage is difficult to obtain.

46. Before contemplating providing a detailed reference on a former employee, it would be important to consider which of the following?

    1. You should check the requirements of the Human Resources Department of your employer.

    2. If the comments are perceived as negative, and the former employee becomes aware of them, you could subject yourself to suit for defamation.

    3. If the employee exhibits unsafe client care practices, it may be wiser to risk legal action from the employee than to subject future clients to this unsafe practitioner.

    4. All of the above.

47. The primary purpose of a pre-employment physical is:

    1. Identify existing health problems that might adversely affect the company's insurance rates.

    2. Determine the mental status of the applicant.

    3. Determine if the applicant is physically capable of doing the job.

    4. Document any existing disabilities and recommend accommodations.

48. A nurse practitioner involved in work-related surveillance knows that the records related to this activity must be held for how many years after employment?

    1. 5 years.

    2. 25 years.

    3. 30 years.

    4. Can be destroyed only after the employee's death.

49. The nurse practitioner knows that, when treating a work-related injury, it is required that he/she:

1. Document thoroughly because of the high probability of legal action.

2. Communicate directly with the client's employer.

3. File a report with the industrial commission documenting the injury and treatment.

4. Notify the Occupational Safety and Health Administration.

50. Which situation would be considered reportable under the Occupational Safety Health Act?

1. A 3-cm abrasion of the forearm.

2. A warehouse worker with back strain reassigned to office work for a week.

3. A twisted ankle that responded to ice and Ace wrap.

4. A minor closed head injury with no loss of consciousness.

51. The purpose of an Occupational Safety and Health Administration 200 log is to record:

1. Occupational injuries and illnesses.

2. Only work-related deaths.

3. Dangerous workplace situations.

4. Lost work days.

52. The Americans with Disabilities Act (ADA) regulates how employers treat the disabled. Under the ADA, disability is defined as a physical or mental impairment that substantially limits one or more major life activities of an individual or a record of a situation in which an individual is regarded as having such an impairment. This would include:

1. A history of addiction.

2. Paralysis.

3. Bipolar disorder.

4. All of the above.

# 21 Answers & Rationales

1. **(2)** The most important advantage of an occurrence policy is that, assuming the policy is in effect at the time of the occurrence, the coverage is available regardless of how long it takes to become aware of a claim (the long "tail" of a medical malpractice claim). The limits do not automatically increase. The carrier need not be notified during the policy period, as is required with claims-made coverage. The coverage under each policy may be as broad as the carrier allows.

2. **(2)** Fact witnesses and necessary paperwork are always easier to discover the closer in time you seek them after a medical misadventure. Memories are fresh and documents are less likely to be misplaced or destroyed. There is no rigid reporting window required by insurance carriers; they do want to be notified in a timely manner. Insurance premiums may be reduced if an insured's track record is clean (i.e., no claims), but not by mere compliance with policy requirements. Risk management employees prefer early notification so that damage control efforts may be implemented promptly, not for regulatory reasons.

3. **(2)** Assessment skills are presumed to be within the purview of the professional nurse, not those with fewer years of nursing education. Also, in this scenario, the LPN is an unknown entity to the delegator. Delegating to the LPN should be done cautiously after determining that person's skill level. Your license is not in jeopardy if you delegated appropriately, as in Option #1, but an error was made and is attributed to the delegatee. Activities in Options #3 and #4 are appropriate for the role.

4. **(4)** Assisted suicide is still a criminal activity in most states (and in legal limbo in the others). Circumventing the client may seem to be an appealing option, but it substitutes paternalism for the autonomy we all claim as our due. A diagnosis of depression can hardly be made with inadequate data; the necessary information can only be determined by conferring with the client herself.

5. **(2)** MCOs are one group of health care organizations impacted by this law. All subscribers must be provided with the stated information at the time of enrollment. Advance directive documents, though extremely helpful in the health care setting, are never mandatory.

6. **(4)** These are the basic requirements for conducting research at health care facilities.

7. **(3)** Your insurance carrier is thoroughly familiar with the processes of handling a claim. They will assist you with every step of this fearsome activity; the first significant obligation they will meet is to put you in touch with your lawyer. Conferring with the client or the client's lawyer is never a wise move. Your colleagues can only offer moral support at this stage; your lawyer is the professional of choice at this time. Never, never even think about altering a record; it can turn a defensible case into a nondefensible one.

8. **(3)** Lobbying for underserved clients is an example of justice, which is the duty to treat all clients fairly, without regard to age, socioeconomic status, or other

variables. Autonomy is the client's right to self-determination without outside control. Nonmaleficence is the duty to prevent or avoid doing harm, whether intentional or unintentional. Veracity is the duty to tell the truth.

9. **(4)** These are all valid reasons to protect your assets in the event of litigation. There is an opposing view regarding the need for professional liability insurance. Some professionals feel that, if there are few assets to protect, insurance is an unnecessary expense. Nurses with professional liability coverage ("deep pockets") could be retained as defendants in a case for a longer period of time.

.0. **(1)** Look to state law to define the circumstances under which confidential medical information may be disclosed. There may be additional requirements imposed by federal regulations (e.g., the handling of certain psychiatric records), but the bulk of the rule-making on this issue is accomplished at the state level. There are exceptions to the requirement of client consent, such as communicable disease reporting to public health authorities and court-ordered record production. Third-party payors, although powerful with their fiscal controls, must produce some proof of client consent to acquire records. An AIDS diagnosis does not shield a record from production, although many states have enacted extra levels of protection for this information. Again, knowledge of state laws is helpful.

.1. **(3)** The ADA does not protect this group of people. In fact, employers may test for illegal drug use; this is not considered a medical examination, which ordinarily is subject to specific requirements under the law.

.2. **(4)** The crux of a bioethical dilemma is that the proposed solution(s) are not perfect, and therefore create some aspect of moral conflict.

.3. **(1)** Callahan believes that health care priorities need to be re-evaluated. He advocates spending first on chronic care

(those who cannot be cured), then preventive care, and lastly on the high-cost, high-tech modalities that benefit few but consume enormous resources.

14. **(2)** The best immediate solution is to identify the item and remove it from service to avoid further client injury. Then, the risk manager, in consultation with the facility's attorneys and/or insurers, will determine how to proceed with equipment analysis. Returning the item to the manufacturer removes it from your control and diminishes your opportunity to defend against a charge of user error. Immediate repair may fail to uncover the real cause of the client injury and impair a successful defense of a claim. If the litigation potential is high, the parties may wish to pool their efforts (and costs) to conduct a third-party review of the equipment. If litigation is likely, then it is also likely that the manufacturer and others in the distribution chain will be co-defendants with the facility and its staff.

15. **(2)** The level of education preferred is that of an advanced degree. The legal issues are the province of the attorneys and the judge; the nurse is expected to be the expert in the clinical issues. Published authorship on nursing issues can add credibility, but specific work experience coupled with the educational credentials are minimally required.

16. **(3)** The APA describes the workings of federal agencies. The PSDA deals with advance directives, and the OBRA '87 changed the rules dealing with long-term care.

17. **(4)** These and other elements combine to produce a program of systematic risk identification, analysis, treatment, and evaluation, with the overall goal of loss prevention.

18. **(4)** Liability insurance is acquired to protect the organization from suits by clients arising from negligent acts of employees. Business interruption coverage is usually purchased in tandem with fire insurance. It reimburses an organization for losses sustained while the business is partially or completely shut down after a catastrophic event. The organization's management team (CEO and senior staff) is insured against losses based upon business judgment errors through directors and officers coverage. Workers' compensation is the line of coverage that protects employees after on-the-job injuries. It is a no-fault system (negligence is not a factor) that covers employee medical bills and pays a percentage of wages while an employee is unable to work.

19. **(1)** You were driving your personal vehicle, so your own auto insurer is "primary"; that is, it responds first to a loss. Since you were on company business, your injuries were sustained "within the course and scope of your employment," so there is coverage under the employer's workers' compensation policy for your medical bills and wage replacement. Depending on the circumstances and policy definitions, there could be some "excess" or additional coverage available under the employer's auto policy, but in no event would that carrier be primarily responsible for your losses. This is not the type of incident that homeowner's insurance is intended to cover. The semi, presumably in use as a business vehicle, would not be insured under a driver's personal auto policy.

20. **(1)** At this point, the mandatory reporting affects only dentists and doctors. Other licensed practitioners are subject to permissive reporting.

21. **(3)** The forwarding facility needs to know whether the receiving facility has space for the new arrival and, more importantly, the ability to treat the particular illness for which the client needs therapy. A familiar example of a client transfer is that of the burn victim, for whom specialty care is mandatory and the locations of that specialty care are usually limited.

22. **(1)** Health care policy within the states is codified or enacted into law by the respective states' legislatures. The boards have significant input (hopefully) in the process, providing the research data and expert "testimony" that the legislatures need in order to make informed decisions. Nursing organizations should also be willing to provide background information and nurse experts to educate the lawmakers.

23. **(3)** The MCOs' cost-containment strategy is enhanced if providers practice within the treatment guidelines suggested by the plans. Providers who inform clients that a certain treatment regimen is the preferred alternative create difficulties if that alternative is excluded from coverage. MCOs usually clearly set out the exclusions in the plan documents, and member services personnel are expected to be able to explain the coverage to subscribers. Experimental treatment, if excluded, would be listed as such in the plan documents.

24. **(2)** These are three of the agencies required to report. Events occurring in the other settings are exempt from reporting requirements under this federal law.

25. **(2)** This is the most factual note; the writer does not apportion blame or assume liability. The other notes would be "red flags" for a chart reviewer. The mention of an incident report makes it virtually impossible to protect these documents from disclosure, especially in those jurisdictions that still afford some protection to these internal early warning documents that seek to alert risk management personnel to a potential claim.

26. **(3)** Clients are often unable to evaluate the quality of the care they receive, but they do react to the way in which the care is delivered. Perceptions by clients of rudeness or "uncaring" on the part of the provider often spur clients to pursue legal action. Clients tend to be more forgiving of less-than-optimal outcomes if they have been involved in the process and are treated with respect.

27. **(4)** Making one's own decisions is the basis for informed consent and the ethical underpinning of the Patient Self-Determination Act. Doing good (Option #1), and its corollary avoiding harm (Option #3),

are ethics principles usually cited as the bases for other health care activities, such as maintaining professional competency. Respect for persons is a more global ethical principle supporting much of a nurse's personal philosophy of caring.

8. **(3)** Usually phrased as duty, breach, proximate cause, and damages, these are the four elements of proof required to prevail in a medical negligence action. Intentional acts are not synonymous with negligent acts. Duty presumes a professional relationship and obligation to provide services. The breach is the error or mistake ascribed to the provider that results in the harm to the client.

9. **(1)** Lay jurors are not expected to know the clinical facts and circumstances involved in a professional negligence claim. The expert witness is necessary to educate the jurors about those medical facts and to testify to the standard of care to be applied. Witnesses with direct involvement in the case are no less credible because of their involvement; their testimony, and personal bias, if any, will be evaluated by the jurors in the context of their roles.

0. **(4)** With respect to nursing specialties, the standard of care is usually a national one. Facility policies, books, and journals are important to review, and physician input may be sought. In some cases, physicians may even be allowed to testify about the standard of care.

1. **(3)** One particular advantage of ADR is the flexibility of the system. In mediation, for example, the mediator can assist with crafting a solution package that meets all the needs of a party, including such things as an apology from the health care provider. Money is not always the only answer. Insurers' goals, however, usually do focus on cash: avoiding huge damage awards to plaintiffs. If a mediator is successful in facilitating case settlements, the costs are usually significantly lower than the costs of a court trial. Insurers with an eye on the bottom line are not averse to these advantages.

2. **(1)** Statutes of limitation set out each state's rules for the timing of the filing of

lawsuits, including malpractice actions. These statutes are procedural laws, in that they describe the "how-to" parameters within which legal rights may be exercised. Minority is considered a legal disability; other state laws usually define it and describe its effects. Rights to sue are not governed by statutes of limitations.

33. **(3)** Statutes may indeed differ from state to state with respect to the breadth of the protection, but most will protect a nurse who renders aid, without expectation of compensation, in a competent manner. Gross negligence will usually void the statutory protections.

34. **(1)** A professional appearance boosts your credibility as a witness. Inappropriate attire and gum-chewing detract from the professional demeanor that you will want to project. Preparation is critical before your words are recorded and transcribed as part of the official litigation transcript. Review documents as noted, but refrain from bringing any materials with you to the deposition without your attorney's approval. Always ask for clarification of ambiguous questions. Speculation is not appropriate. Your professional work history is always asked, so a copy of your curriculum vitae (CV) is a useful tool to bring along to a deposition.

35. **(1)** Jousting in the client's medical record is never a good idea. It provides fodder for plaintiff's lawyers but does not contribute to quality nursing care. If you have a conflict with another provider, deal with the provider directly, preferably in person. Another arena for resolving such disputes is the quality review process.

36. **(4)** All of these factors enter into an analysis of whether it is appropriate to accept a minor's consent to treatment. Another factor to consider is the type of treatment sought. Some states have statutes allowing minors to consent to specific therapies, such as treatment for venereal disease.

37. **(4)** Long-term care is a specialized area with layers of regulatory requirements, most stemming from the federal government. Nurses who work in this environment need to be vigilant about learning the rules and maintaining compliance. Ongoing, effective communication with regulators is essential.

38. **(4)** We have a tendency to get very careless with our information management and the way we interact with clients and their very personal data. The often wide-open and very frantic front-desk atmosphere of an office does little to calm client fears that their information will be too-easily accessible to those without a need to know.

39. **(2)** Sexual preference is not a protected classification. The other options refer to different federal laws that provide varying degrees of protection to those groups. It is prudent to check with your business attorney to determine if the policies you have drafted for your office are in compliance with federal guidelines. The Equal Employment Opportunity Commission (EEOC), which enforces the laws, publishes guidelines about the various statutes. These publications are available, either free or at minimal cost, from the agency. Some may be available on the Internet.

40. **(3)** This seems to fit the criteria for a hostile environment, a form of sexual harassment. The harassment seems to be pervasive and longstanding; the women have complained and apparently no action has been taken. The isolated incident and single data request do not rise to the level of harassment. The participants did not find the actions objectionable, and job performance was not affected. In Option #2, although the potential was there for the nurse to use the prior relationship as a club to either downgrade the employee or deny a benefit, this result did not occur.

41. **(1)** This is the overall goal of the ADA. It is not another entitlement program, and it cannot impose wheelchair ramp requirements on every building owner in America. Access ramps and interpreters may be required as a "reasonable accommodation" to qualified people in certain defined circumstances. There is no across-the-board mandate for these types of aid to the handicapped.

42. **(1)** The Supreme Court essentially deferred to the states to legislate on this topic. In most states, the activity is not permitted. In one of the states involved, in the high court's case, a statute permitting assisted suicide is being challenged. Nurse practitioners need to look at their states' laws on this topic for guidance. The other providers referenced in Options #2, #3, and #4 would act at their peril if their states' laws followed the current majority view.

43. **(1)** The purpose of a medical malpractice action is to make the claimant whole by the awarding of money damages. The award compensates the claimant or plaintiff for the wrong (or tort) he has suffered at the hands of the defendant. On the criminal side, the state sues on behalf of society for violations of society's criminal laws. The punishment is fines, imprisonment, or both. Professional liability insurance usually excludes criminal and intentional acts, so coverage for these types of activities is unlikely.

44. **(4)** The full-blown jury trial is what ADR seeks to avoid. Mediation and arbitration are the most well-known forms of ADR. Some jurisdictions use the settlement conference as a technique to attempt settlement after a lawsuit has been filed but before a trial begins. Another type of ADR is called a summary jury trial, which is a private, shortened version wherein the parties share some evidence and get a sense of the strengths and weaknesses of each side's position. There are also hybrids such as "med-arb," wherein a proceeding starts out as a mediation but, if the case does not settle, it is referred to an arbitrator for resolution.

45. **(3)** This is the so-called long tail of professional liability; there is always a time lag from the date of injury to the date a claimant files a malpractice action. In the case of an infant, that time lag can be many years because of the effect of the statute of limitations. This extends the period of potential risk to the nurse who cares for children. Although there may be a sympathy factor involved when jurors decide damages awards, the judgment is

usually proportional to the injury and not the age of the claimant. Insurance coverage for pediatric providers is no less available than for other specialties; insurers adjust premiums to account for the level of risk.

6. **(4)** If the Human Resources Department has established guidelines for the handling of references, it would be wise to follow them. It is also an effective mechanism to deflect potentially problematic queries by passing requests to the department most equipped to handle them. Most employers will be very circumspect about the information released, often limiting the data to dates of employment only. Absent some protective state legislation, employers should be prudent about sharing comments on former employees' work histories.

7. **(3)** The purpose is to determine the appropriateness of the applicant for the job. Identifying health problems to prevent hiring an individual is discriminatory. The mental status and disabilities may also be a part of the pre-employment physical but are not the primary purpose.

48. **(3)** The Occupational Safety and Health Administration requires that these records be held for 30 years after termination of employment.

49. **(3)** It is required by law that a report of any work-related injury be filed with the industrial commission of the state in which the injury occurred.

50. **(2)** The Occupational Safety and Health Administration requires the report of any injury or illness that requires more than first aid treatment and/or involves loss of work time, limited work status, loss of consciousness, or death.

51. **(1)** The purpose is to record occupational injuries and illnesses, which would also include death reports and lost work days and would also reveal dangerous working conditions.

52. **(4)** All of the conditions listed would qualify under the ADA and may require accommodation in the workplace.